EATING FOR AUTISM

EATING FOR AUTISM

THE 10-STEP NUTRITION PLAN
TO HELP TREAT
YOUR CHILD'S AUTISM,
ASPERGER'S, OR ADHD

Elizabeth Strickland, MS, RD, LD
with Suzanne McCloskey
Recipes by Roben Ryberg

Da Capo
LIFE
LONG

A MEMBER OF THE PERSEUS BOOKS GROUP

Copyright © 2009 by Elizabeth Strickland, Suzanne McCloskey, and Roben Ryberg

Composition and design in 11.5 Garamond by Cynthia Young.

Library of Congress Cataloging-in-Publication Data
Strickland, Elizabeth, 1956–
Eating for autism : the 10-step nutrition plan to help treat your child's autism, Asperger's, or
    ADHD / Elizabeth Strickland with Suzanne McCloskey ; recipes by Roben Ryberg.
        p. cm.
    Includes bibliographical references and index.
    ISBN 978-0-7382-1243-2
    1. Autism in children—Diet therapy.   2. Asperger's syndrome in children—Diet
    therapy.   3. Attention-deficit hyperactivity disorder—Diet therapy.   I. McCloskey,
    Suzanne.   II. Ryberg, Roben.   III. Title.
RJ506.A9S775 2009
618.92'858820654—dc22

                                                                                        2009001366

First Da Capo Press edition 2009

Published by Da Capo Press
A Member of the Perseus Books Group
www.dacapopress.com

Da Capo Press books are available at special discounts for bulk purchases in the U.S. by corporations, institutions, and other organizations. For more information, please contact the Special Markets Department at the Perseus Books Group, 2300 Chestnut Street, Suite 200, Philadelphia, PA, 19103, or call (800) 810-4145, ext. 5000, or e-mail special.markets@perseusbooks.com.

10 9 8 7 6 5

This book is dedicated to my children Jacob, Jessica, and Jackson.
I carry each of you in my heart. Thanks for sharing your mom
over the years and making it possible for me to
help so many other children.

CONTENTS

PART III: NUTRITIONAL INFORMATION

PREFACE

Since earning my bachelor's degree in dietetics and my master's degree in nutrition twenty-five years ago, I've spent my professional career providing nutrition therapy to children who suffer from all kinds of health issues—from developmental disabilities, metabolic disorders, and gastrointestinal disorders to food allergies, feeding problems, and chronic illness. During this time, I've seen a dramatic and encouraging shift in the public's perception of nutrition. People are taking more personal responsibility for their health and the health of their children. Parents are becoming increasingly proactive about safeguarding their children's health. They are questioning the overuse of medication and searching for safer, effective, natural alternatives. They're beginning to understand that healthy foods, nutrients, vitamins, minerals, antioxidants, amino acids, essential fatty acids, herbs, and nutraceuticals play a huge role in maintaining their children's health and supporting their ability to heal.

Now the bad news—I've also seen an alarming increase in the rate of many serious health conditions, such as autism, Attention Deficit Disorder (ADD), Attention Deficit Hyperactivity Disorder (ADHD), learning disabilities, asthma, food allergies, and obesity in our children. Twenty-five years ago, autism was rare; now 1 in 150 children are diagnosed with the disorder. ADD and ADHD are sweeping the country, with more than 2 million children diagnosed. Between 5 and 10 percent of schoolchildren are diagnosed with learning disabilities. Asthma is reaching epidemic proportions, affecting more than 6 percent of kids in the United States. More than 12 million children and adults suffer from food allergies, and the numbers continue to rise.

I was particularly moved by the rising rate of autism in our kids, and about fifteen years ago, I began to focus my practice on treating kids with the condition, as well as related disorders such as Asperger's Syndrome, Pervasive Developmental Disorder–Not Otherwise Specified (PDD-NOS), ADD, and ADHD. First identified in 1943 by Dr. Leo Kanner of Johns Hopkins University, autism remains the most puzzling childhood disorder. To this day, no one knows what causes autism, how best to treat it, and why some kids recover while others do not. This means that treating autism is literally like putting together the pieces of a puzzle. There is no "cookie cutter" approach. Every child is unique and responds to a different variety of treatment approaches. Therefore it's critical that you work together with your child's medical team to create the most effective combination of therapies for your child.

Treatment of autism typically includes medication, special education services, behavioral programs, occupational therapy, sensory integration therapy, speech-language therapy, complementary and alternative medicine (CAM), biomedical treatment, and numerous other therapies such as art, music, and **hippotherapy**. However, too often there's one critical element missing—nutrition therapy.

The right nutritional interventions can have a huge impact on your child's brain function, memory, learning, attention, focus, mood, behavior, growth, and overall health. Nutrition can protect your child's body from neurotoxins, enhance his immune system, and support his gastrointestinal function. Unfortunately, many physicians and other healthcare professionals don't recognize the importance of nutrition therapy in treating autism and even discourage parents from pursuing nutritional interventions. I believe this happens in large part because of the false claims that have been made that a special diet or nutritional supplement can "cure" autism or create "miraculous recoveries." I also think part of the problem lies in the massive amount of controversial and questionable information about nutritional interventions used to treat autism found on the Internet. Sadly, there are many unqualified people out there claiming to be nutritionists who provide parents with misinformation, false claims, and testimonials and sell them all kinds of ineffective and costly nutritional supplements.

The truth is, no diet or supplement will miraculously cure autism. However, you *can* use food, supplements, herbs, and nutraceuticals to feed your autistic child's starving brain and body and maximize his brain function, which will make him more responsive to other treatments and therapies. Nutrition is the basis upon which all other treatments are built, and nutrition therapy should be a part of every autistic child's comprehensive treatment plan.

I wrote this book because I want to help both parents and professionals better understand the role of nutrition therapy in treating autism, Asperger's, PDD-NOS, ADD, and ADHD. Unlike other books on these conditions, which dedicate at best one chapter to nutritional interventions, *Eating for Autism* is focused solely on nutrition. I've spent many years treating hundreds of children with these conditions, and I've gained a very clear understanding of parents' concerns, questions, and specific needs for help regarding nutrition. *Eating for Autism* is specifically designed for:

Parents who are seeking guidance in making informed decisions about safe and effective nutritional interventions for their children. It's my hope that this book will help you separate fact from fiction with regard to the information on nutritional interventions found on the Internet and suggested by some practitioners. I encourage you to use this book when discussing nutritional interventions with your child's physician, dietitian, educators, and other healthcare professionals.

Registered dietitians who are seeking to enhance their clinical skills in providing nutrition therapy to children with autism. There's new and controversial information about nutrition interventions constantly emerging in the autism community. Dietitians are obligated to research and evaluate new proposed nutritional interventions and provide families with reliable information so they can make safe, responsible decisions regarding diets, supplements, and nutrition therapy for their children.

Physicians who would like to know more about the critical role nutrition therapy plays in the comprehensive treatment of autism. When physicians emphasize the role that nutrition plays in enhancing a child's brain and body function, it encourages parents to take good nutrition more seriously. Physicians can also refer parents to a registered dietitian who specializes in developmental disabilities.

Educators who are seeking a broader understanding of how nutrition impacts children's cognitive function and their ability to learn in the classroom. It's critical for educators to understand how certain foods, food additives, and nutrient deficiencies contribute to behavioral problems, hyperactivity, inattentiveness, and poor classroom performance. Nutritional interventions can help children with autism benefit from their special education services and should be considered in the educational system.

Other healthcare professionals who want to understand why nutrition therapy is an important component to treating autism. If an autistic child is nutritionally compromised, it will negatively impact his ability to respond to other treatment approaches, such as behavioral programs and art, music, hippo-, occupational, sensory integration, and speech-language therapies. All therapists involved in treating autism should advocate for the inclusion of nutrition therapy, so these children are better able to benefit from their treatment approaches.

Eating for Autism will give you the tools you need to make nutrition therapy an effective part of your child's autism treatment and improve both his functioning and his well-being.

Note: I've kept the medical jargon to a minimum, but you may run into some terms you're not familiar with. For your convenience, terms that appear in **boldface** indicate that they're defined in the glossary on page 241.

ACKNOWLEDGMENTS

Many very talented people helped me with this book, and I would like to express my appreciation for their time and effort. First, I would like to thank Sue McCloskey for her hours of hard work on this project, Roben Ryberg for creating delicious child and family friendly gluten-free, casein-free recipes, and Steve Cooley for designing such a beautiful book cover. I also would like to express my appreciation to everyone at Da Capo Lifelong Books, especially Katie McHugh, for supporting this project.

I would like to express my special thanks and gratitude to the children and parents I've had the privilege to serve over the past twenty-five years. They have been a personal inspiration to me. I am constantly in awe of their strength and determination.

For my mom, dad, brothers Philip and Wayne, and sisters Patricia and Bonnie for their continued support and interest in my career over the years.

And special heartfelt thanks to Keith Sauls, who provided me with constant encouragement, support, and laughs throughout the entire process of writing this book. Keith, thank you for bringing so much love and happiness into my life!

Thank you!

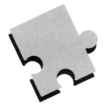

INTRODUCTION

Understanding the Autism-Nutrition Connection

Most people, including healthcare professionals, don't put much thought into food or nutrition. When they think about food, it's usually about how it tastes, looks, smells, or feels in their mouths. Typically the focus of family gatherings, holidays, and parties, food gives us a reason to get together and socialize. We don't often stop to consider what it actually does in our bodies. But when you have a child with autism or a related disorder, it's critical to understand that food is more than just something that brings us pleasure. What your child eats can have a major positive or negative impact on his brain and bodily functions. Therefore, it's important for you to know exactly how food impacts your child. Both you and your child's healthcare team need to recognize that without proper nutrition, your child will not function at his full potential and will not fully benefit from his therapy sessions. Following are just a few examples how a poor diet can negatively affect your child:

Brain development and function. Your child's brain is highly dependent on the vitamins, minerals, amino acids, essential fatty acids, and calories found in food. For instance, if your child is not getting enough of certain key nutrients, it compromises his **neurotransmitter** production, the synthesis of his brain's **myelin sheath**, **glucose oxidation**, and his visual and cognitive processing. If he's consuming too much sugar and artificial additives, it can compromise his brain function and contribute to behavior and learning problems.

Detoxification processes. Your child must consume zinc, selenium, magnesium, beta carotene, vitamin A, vitamin E, and choline to help his liver naturally rid his body of harmful neurotoxins like mercury, lead, arsenic, cadmium, dioxins, PCBs, pesticides, and solvents. Exposure to these neurotoxins can damage your child's brain and **central**

1

nervous system, which in turn could cause him to have a lower IQ, learning disabilities, attention deficit, hyperactivity, impulsivity, compulsive behavior, aggression, violence, speech difficulties, memory impairment, **motor dysfunction**, developmental delays, and mental retardation.

Gastrointestinal (GI) health. The GI tract is highly dependent on the amino acid glutamine and requires a constant supply of vitamins and minerals for normal bowel function. If your child has nutritional deficiencies, it can impair new cellular growth in his gastrointestinal tract, which in turn compromises his ability to absorb the nutrients he consumes in foods. When this occurs, it makes other nutritional deficiencies that impact the brain and body even worse.

Immune system function. Our immune system relies on vitamin C, vitamin A, vitamin E, vitamin D, B vitamins, iron, selenium, zinc, and bioflavonoids to function at its optimum level. A poor diet puts your child at greater risk for developing allergies as well as frequent ear infections, acute and chronic illnesses, and upper respiratory infections. If your child is continually fighting off illness, he will inevitably miss school and therapy sessions, which will further compromise his response to treatment.

Erythropoiesis. Erythropoiesis is the process by which red blood cells are produced, usually in the bone marrow. Red blood cells are the vehicles that transport oxygen to our brains and throughout our bodies. Key nutrients that support this process include iron, vitamin B_6, copper, folate, vitamin B_{12}, vitamin C, and vitamin E. Dietary deficiencies in these nutrients can cause anemia, which can lead to irritability, headaches, loss of appetite, lethargy, hyperactivity, inattentiveness, and poor school performance.

Nutritional Problems are Common with Autism. A large percentage of children with autism, Asperger's, PDD-NOS, ADD, and ADHD struggle with one or more of the following nutritional problems:

- poor diet
- nutritional deficiencies
- feeding problems
- food allergies
- food intolerances
- chemical sensitivities
- gastrointestinal disorders
- exposure to neurotoxins
- frequent illnesses and infections
- negative drug and nutrient interactions

 Children with autism also often have dysfunctional immune systems and inadequate detoxification processes. These nutritional problems place a huge burden on your child and are slowly eating away at his health and ability to function to his highest potential. In fact, I'm amazed that many kids with autism and nutritional problems are able to function at all, much less go to school, sit still, focus, process information, learn, and participate in therapy sessions. *Eating for Autism* will show you how to relieve your child of these nutritional burdens. You'll see that as each of your child's nutritional problems is treated and resolved, his health and behavior will improve. Your child will function better and respond better to all facets of his treatment.

NUTRITIONAL INTERVENTIONS USED TO TREAT AUTISM

If you've already begun investigating nutritional interventions as a way to help treat your child's autism, you probably know that there are many different ones out there, such as restrictive diets, high-dose vitamins, supplements, and more. What you may not know is that specific nutritional interventions are usually designed to target specific issues a child may have, such as improving cognitive functioning, or treating physical problems like food allergies, GI disorders, and immune and detoxification system dysfunction. Here's a list of the most common nutrition interventions used in the autism community:

Diets
- Gluten Free Casein Free
- Elimination/Challenge
- Specific Carbohydrate Diet (SCD)
- Rotation
- Antifungal
- Feingold

Basic Nutrition Supplements
- multivitamins and minerals
- essential fatty acids

High-Dose Vitamins
- vitamin B_6

Nutrients, Herbs, and Nutraceuticals

probiotics

antifungals

digestive enzymes

amino acids

dimethylglycine (DMG)

trimethylglycine (TMG)

coenzyme Q_{10}

phosphatidylcholine

bioflavonoids

proanthocyandins

N-acetyl-cysteine (NAC)

alpha-lipoic acid (ALA)

antioxidants

pyridoxal 5 phosphate (P5P)

carnosine

carnitine

glutathione

vitamin B_{12}

Many of these nutritional interventions are controversial, and the medical community doesn't encourage parents to try them because there's little science-based research available on them. In fact, most of the current research on nutritional interventions to treat autism is anecdotal, which means it's based on nonscientific observations or studies. In the medical world, only double-blind, randomized, placebo-controlled clinical trials can prove the effectiveness of a proposed nutrition theory (i.e., Can a gluten-free, casein-free diet improve autistic symptoms?). There are several reasons for this lack of scientific evidence in the area of nutritional interventions:

Scientific studies are extremely difficult to perform. Getting approval for and performing human studies, especially on children with developmental disabilities, is a huge challenge. A scientific study on the effectiveness of a gluten-free, casein-free diet, for example, would require gathering together a group of hundreds of children diagnosed with autism and making sure all of their treatment approaches remained consistent while changing just one variable—their diet. The study would need to be conducted blindly, without the children, parents, therapists, and investigators knowing which group of children in the study are on the diet and which are not. The complexity of conducting this kind of scientific-based research study is prohibitive, so anecdotal-based research is conducted instead.

Research in the area of autism is fairly new. It was only in December 2006 that the U.S. government finally recognized autism as a national problem and authorized $1 billion of federal funding for autism-related research. However, conducting science-based research studies takes time. It could take another ten or even twenty years for the medical community to agree on the interpretation of the results of these studies and apply them in the real world of treating children with autism. If you have a child diagnosed with autism today, that's simply too long for you to wait.

Funding is scarce. Lack of private and federal funding is the primary reason why so few science-based research studies have been conducted on nutritional interventions. Of the $1 billion the federal government has made available for autism research, *none* of it is designated for nutritional interventions research. As long as funding for research on nutritional interventions remains scarce, lack of scientific evidence will continue to be an issue.

It's important to remember that just because most of the research on nutritional interventions is anecdotal instead of scientific, that doesn't mean that they don't work or shouldn't be considered when creating a treatment plan for autism. Hopefully, adequate funding will become available in the near future that will enable us to conduct science-based research on nutritional interventions that anecdotal evidence suggests is effective in reducing the symptoms of autism. This will help cement nutrition therapy's place as part of mainstream autism treatment.

HOW THIS BOOK CAN HELP YOU

Even the most well-read, technologically savvy parent can become confused and overwhelmed when it comes to nutrition therapy. There's so much information out there on the Internet, passed along in parent support groups and the media, from both medical and non-medical sources—it's difficult to sift through it all. It's next to impossible for parents to analyze the scientific and anecdotal evidence, consider restrictive diets and high-dose vitamins, select an appropriate vitamin/mineral supplement, decide which nutrients, herbs, and nutraceuticals are right for their children, and implement all these nutritional interventions safely without professional help. Even *with* professional help, many parents get so overwhelmed, frustrated, and discouraged that they decide to give up.

Over the last several years, I've developed a ten-step approach to integrating nutritional interventions into treatment plans for children with autism and related disorders. *Eating for Autism* will guide you step-by-step through the process, starting with basic nutritional interventions and gradually moving to more advanced levels of nutrition therapy. My approach is family-friendly and easy to implement, and it allows you to move through each step at your own pace and level of comfort.

This book is designed to be used to suit each reader's individual needs. For instance, you may see a significant improvement in your child after implementing just the basic steps and choose to stop at that point. Or, after mastering the basic steps, you may choose to implement only a few of the advanced steps. Many parents choose to implement every step in the program. (It's important to note that each step builds on the previous one and gets more advanced as the book progresses, so you need to implement them in the order I've provided.) Whether you're just interested in the basic steps or want to apply more advance interventions, you are sure to see positive improvements in your child's condition, from his behavior, mood, sleeping patterns, and overall health to his response to other treatment approaches.

PART I:
THE PLAN

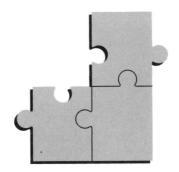

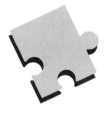

STEP 1

Transition Your Child to a Healthy Diet

One of the biggest mistakes I see parents make when it comes to incorporating nutrition therapy into their children's treatment program is jumping into advanced interventions instead of starting with the basics. In nutrition therapy, each step builds upon the previous one, becoming more advanced as you work your way through the program. The first thing you need to do is identify and resolve any basic nutrition issues your child may have. He won't be able to properly respond to or benefit from advanced nutrition interventions if basic nutrition is still a problem.

Basic nutrition has become a serious issue for our children over the last twenty years because it has changed so dramatically. The food children eat today is nothing like the food children ate in previous generations. Today, children subsist mainly on foods that are highly processed, lacking in nutrients, and loaded with artificial chemicals, preservatives, trans fats, excess sugar, and pesticide residues. Take a look at the ingredients list on some of the packaged foods you have in your refrigerator or pantry. I'll bet the list is a mile long, and you can't even pronounce most of the ingredients, much less know what they are. The repercussions of this shift away from poor nutrition are serious. We've seen a dramatic increase in developmental and neurological disorders in our children. Therefore, step one is to transition your child onto a diet that consists of whole, healthy foods and eliminate all unnecessary artificial ingredients.

ELIMINATE SYNTHETIC FOOD ADDITIVES

There are twenty-four different types of synthetic food additives found in the foods we eat. Before a food additive is added to our foods, it must be deemed **"generally recognized as safe" (GRAS)** and approved by the Food and Drug Administration (FDA). This means that it's been proven safe for the general public and poses no significant health hazard, such as promoting cancer. But the reality is that we are consuming human-made chemicals with virtually every bite of food, and no one really knows what effect they may be having on our immune, respiratory, endocrine, and nervous systems. There's a lot of controversy in the medical community about what the short- and long-term impact of these chemicals may be on a growing child's brain and nervous system. The autism community is particularly concerned about four of the synthetic food additives: artificial colors, artificial flavors, preservatives, and artificial sweeteners.

Here is a list of the twenty-four types of food additives found in the foods we eat:

acidity regulators	flour treatment	seasonings
anti-caking agents	food acids	sequestrants
anti-foaming agents	gelling agents	stabilizers
food coloring	glazing agents	artificial sweeteners
color fixatives	humectants	thickeners
color retention	improving agents	vegetable gums
emulsifiers	mineral salts	
firming agents	preservatives	
flavor enhancers	propellants	

Artificial Colors

There are seven artificial colors currently permitted in our foods in the United States: Blue No. 1, Blue No. 2, Green No. 3, Red No. 40, Red No. 3, Yellow No. 5, and Yellow No. 6. There's a growing body of research that indicates some children are sensitive to these artificial colors and that they aggravate their ADD and ADHD symptoms. Most recently, a study published in the November 2007 issue of *The Lancet* concluded that artificial colors in the diets of children resulted in increased hyperactivity. Research also indicates that ingesting artificial colors may result in behavioral changes such as irritability, restlessness, and sleep disturbance. Other research indicates that when ingested, some artificial colors may aggravate the symptoms of hives, eczema, dermatitis, rhinitis, and asthma. There's an additional issue that many parents are not aware of—most artificial colors are made from a mixture of phenols, polycyclic aromatic hydrocarbons, and heterocyclic compounds called **coal tar**. Coal tar is the by-product of coal when it's carbonized to make coke (a fuel) or gasified to make coal gas. Coal tar is also found in medicated shampoo, soap, and ointments, and is used as a treatment to kill head lice. According to the International Agency for Research on Cancer, any product with a certain percentage of crude coal tar is considered a Group 1 carcinogen. Clearly, too much coal tar is a bad thing. Given all of the possible adverse effects artificial colors can have on your child, I strongly encourage you to remove them from his diet. This step will definitely help relieve your child's physical and behavioral symptoms, though the degree to which it will help will depend on the level of his sensitivity to chemicals.

Artificial Flavors

Artificial flavors are chemically synthesized compounds added to foods to either imitate or enhance a natural flavor. There are approximately seventeen hundred artificial flavors approved by the FDA. An artificial flavor of particular concern in the autism community is **monosodium glutamate (MSG)**. MSG is the sodium salt of an amino acid called glutamic acid and the ionized form of glutamate. It's used commercially as a flavor enhancer and found in many common food products such as canned soups, beef and chicken stocks, flavored potato chips, snack foods, frozen dinners, instant meals with seasoning mixtures, and foods from fast-food restaurants. Some fermented products have naturally occurring glutamate, such as soy sauce, steak sauce, and Worcestershire sauce. Glutamate may also be present in a variety of other additives, such as hydrolyzed vegetable protein, hydrolyzed soy protein, autolyzed yeast, hydrolyzed yeast, yeast extract, soy extracts, and protein isolate.

MSG isn't always easy to spot on a food label. Be on the lookout for the terms "spices" and "natural flavorings" on a food label. They indicate that it may contain MSG. The food additives "disodium inosinate" and "disodium guanylate" are used only with MSG, so if these additives are on a food label, there's a good chance that MSG is also in the food product.

MSG is "generally recognized as safe" by the FDA; however, there *are* health concerns. Glutamic acid is classified as an **excitotoxin**, and animal studies indicate that ingesting a high level of it causes brain damage. While most researchers agree it's unlikely that human adults could ingest enough MSG to create glutamic acid levels high enough to promote neurological damage, there is concern about the unknown long-term neurodegenerative effects of small to moderate rises of glutamic acid in our systems over time. Researchers are also concerned about the potential short- and long-term effects MSG may have on infants and young children. There appears to be a number of people who are sensitive to MSG and develop acute adverse reactions such as headache, facial pressure, chest pain, nausea, difficulty breathing, drowsiness, weakness, and aggravation of asthma symptoms. What if, for example, you have an autistic child who is nonverbal with severe behavioral problems and is sensitive to an artificial flavor like MSG? If he consumes it in his diet on a regular basis and develops a severe headache every day, how is he going to tell you? Since he's nonverbal, he'll communicate to you through his behavior—he may slap himself in the head, head bang, self abuse, become irritable, un-cooperative, or have tantrums. Sensitivity to one or more artificial flavors may be caus-ing or exacerbating a physical problem for your child, which in turn may be causing a behavioral problem. Removing artificial flavors from his diet is a critical step toward im-proving his symptoms.

Artificial Preservatives

A preservative is a natural or human-made chemical that is added to food products to inhibit the growth of bacteria and fungi, inhibit oxidation, and prevent changes in the food's color, odor, and taste. Natural preservatives include salt, sugar, and vinegar, and the processes of freezing, pickling, smoking, and salting are also used to preserve foods naturally. Artificial preservatives are controversial because research has shown that some of them cause various health problems, respiratory problems, and cancer. Re-search also shows that artificial preservatives aggravate ADD and ADHD symptoms in some children.

Artificial preservatives do affect your child. A research study conducted in New York City Public Schools showed that when artificial additives, including preservatives, were eliminated from the school food program, the students' academic performance in-creased and disciplinary problems decreased.

The autism community is particularly concerned about the effect that the artificial preservatives **butylated hydroxytoluene (BHT)** and **butylated hydroxyanisole (BHA)** may have on children. BHT and BHA are fat-soluble phenol compounds ap-proved by the FDA to be used as an antioxidant food additive. They're also used in pharmaceuticals, cosmetics, jet fuels, rubber, petroleum products, and embalming fluid. Research indicates that BHT, which can be found in cereal, chewing gum, and high-fat foods such as potato chips and shortening, promotes certain forms of cancer and tumors. Many countries, such as Japan, Romania, Sweden, and Australia have banned BHT from use in foods, but the United States has not yet followed suit. However, the United States has barred it from being used in baby foods. Many food industries have voluntarily eliminated BHT from their foods and replaced it with the preservative BHA, but there are also serious concerns about BHA. After conducting animal studies, the National Institutes of Health (NIH) concluded that it's reason-able to assume that BHA is a human carcinogen (cancer forming). Researchers also suspect that people with dysfunctional detoxification systems (or whose bodies have trouble eliminating toxins from their system) may have difficulty processing both BHT and BHA. In children with autism, this is expressed as behavioral problems. (Turn to Step 10 for more about the problems a dysfunctional detoxification system can cause for children and why they are more vulnerable to adverse reactions to artificial colors, flavors, and preservatives.) Eliminating artificial preservatives, especially BHT and BHA, from your child's diet should help relieve some of his behavioral symptoms.

Artificial Sweeteners

Artificial sweeteners are human-made compounds that are many times sweeter than **sucrose**, or table sugar. Their safety and potential for health risks, including cancer, has been a longstanding controversy in the medical community. The three most commonly used artificial sweeteners in the United States are **saccharin** (Sweet'N Low), **sucralose** (Splenda), and **aspartame** (NutraSweet and Equal). Saccharin, the first artificial sweetener created, is three hundred to five hundred times sweeter than table sugar. Saccharin is FDA-approved in the United States, but some countries allow only a restricted level of use, and other countries have banned it completely.

Sucralose is a chlorinated sugar that is six hundred times sweeter than table sugar. It belongs to a class of chemicals called **organochlorides**, some of which are highly toxic or carcinogenic. However, many researchers suggest that since sucralose is insoluble in fat, it doesn't accumulate in fat as do other organochlorides, which reduces its risk of toxicity.

The artificial sweetener aspartame is derived from two amino acids, **aspartic acid** and **phenylalanine**, and is two hundred times sweeter than table sugar. While animal research indicates that aspartame may cause brain cancer in rats, other research shows that it doesn't cause cancer in humans. However, headaches and seizures have been reported in relation to aspartame, making its safety a much-debated topic. In the autism community, the focus is on the impact aspartame may have on a child's brain function. Normally, food contains a variety of amino acids, so after your child consumes a food, his brain receives a balanced combination of several amino acids. But when he drinks an aspartame-sweetened drink, which is heavily concentrated with only two amino acids, his brain receives a sudden dose of only two amino acids. This unnatural influx disrupts the sensitive balance among neurotransmitters in the brain and may result in neurological problems. Many believe that when children with autism experience this neurotransmitter imbalance, it results in mood and behavioral problems that aggravate their current behavioral symptoms.

Until recently, the food industry had been using corn syrup as a low-cost alternative to sugar in products that traditionally contain sugar. Now, artificial sweeteners are being used to replace both sugar *and* corn syrup, making it the more cost effective choice for food manufacturers.

Though all of these artificial sweeteners are approved for use by the FDA, there's still much debate surrounding their long-term safety, especially for children who could potentially have decades of continued exposure. It's important to understand that just because a food additive has been approved by the FDA as GRAS, this doesn't necessarily mean it's safe for our children. Aspartame is a perfect example of this fact. I urge you to be cautious and eliminate all artificial sweeteners from your child's diet.

Jason ate a pretty good variety of foods, but I knew they were all unhealthy and lacking in nutrition. Honestly, his diet wasn't a priority for me at that time because I was so overwhelmed dealing with his diagnosis and behavioral problems and trying to find therapies to help him. After attending Elizabeth's seminar on nutrition and autism, I had a much better understanding of how Jason's diet and the artificial chemicals in the foods he ate could affect his brain, behavior, and ability to function normally. I started gradually replacing the foods he ate with foods free of artificial colors, flavors, and excess sugar. I purchased fewer prepackaged foods and started cooking more meals from scratch using "real" food. Just making these few changes in Jason's diet made a big difference. He became less aggressive, stopped hitting and kicking me, and became a calmer, more pleasant child.

—*Mother of Jason, a seven-year-old with ADHD*

LIMIT FOODS THAT CONTAIN TRANS FAT

Trans fat is the product of **hydrogenation**, which is the process by which hydrogen is added to liquid vegetable oil. The fatty acids in the oil then acquire some of the hydrogen, which makes it denser. Typically, the hydrogenation process is only partially completed in order to produce a more malleable fat that is solid at room temperature but will melt upon baking. **Partially hydrogenated** fats have replaced natural solid fats and natural liquid oils in our foods because they're cheaper to use than the real thing, and they prolong the shelf life and flavor stability of foods. When you start reading food labels, you may be astonished by the number of products that contain partially hydrogenated oils and therefore trans fat. Trans fat can be found in vegetable shortenings, some margarines, crackers, cookies, chips, cakes, pies, bread, snack foods, and foods fried in partially hydrogenated oils. It's also used in some dietary supplements, energy bars, and nutrition bars. In January 2006, the FDA required food manufacturers to list trans fat on their product labels. Dietary supplement manufacturers are also required to list trans fat on the product label if it contains more than 0.5 grams.

Many people don't know that trans fat also occurs naturally in the milk and body fat of certain animals, such as cows and sheep. According to the U.S. National Dairy Council, these natural trans fats found in animal foods don't appear to have the same negative effects as human-made hydrogenated oils.

There are a number of reasons why we should all stay away from trans fats. They raise our LDL (bad cholesterol) and lower our HDL (good cholesterol), which increases our risk of coronary heart disease. There's also growing concern that trans fats may increase our risk for cancer, type 2 diabetes, obesity, and infertility. But the autism community is especially interested in the negative impact trans fat has on the liver. Trans fats interfere with the enzyme **delta 6 desaturase**, which is critical in the process of converting **essential fatty acids** (also known as omega-3 and omega-6 fatty acids) found in foods to the active forms (arachidonic acid [ARA], eicosapentaenoic acid [EPA], and docosahexaenoic acid [DHA]) used by the brain. A deficiency of delta 6 desaturase causes a deficiency of ARA, EPA, and DHA, which are critical for brain development, brain function, brain cell signaling, and vision processing. Research indicates that children diagnosed with ADD, ADHD, dyslexia, dyspraxia, and autism may already have low levels of delta 6 desaturase, so when these children consume foods with trans fat, it makes their situations worse. (Turn to Step 4 for more information on how a delta 6 desaturase deficiency can affect your child.) I strongly encourage you to keep the trans fat in your child's diet to a minimum.

You can find omega-3 fatty acids in fish, flaxseed oil, canola oil, walnuts, and pumpkin seeds. Omega-6 fatty acids can be found in soy oil, corn oil, safflower oil, evening primrose oil, borage oil, and black currant seed oil.

STAY AWAY FROM HIGHLY PROCESSED FOODS

Most families live a pretty fast-paced lifestyle these days, and finding time to prepare home-cooked meals made with fresh whole foods can be difficult. Instead, more and more families depend on the convenience of pre-packaged foods and fast foods. Unfortunately, we're paying a very high price for the sake of convenience. A generation ago, a "processed" meal simply meant cleaning fresh foods and basic kitchen preparation. Back then, foods contained a higher percentage of their original vitamins, minerals, phytonutrients, and fiber. The highly processed foods we depend on today have a lower nutritional value; are higher in fat, salt, and sugar; and contain trans fat and many food additives that may contribute to behavioral and health problems. Sit-down family meals prepared from scratch have become virtually obsolete. I believe that the best way to limit these unhealthy, processed foods from your child's diet (and your entire family's diet) is to make family meals a priority in your home. Here's some advice to help make this happen:

- Buy one or two cookbooks with recipes to prepare healthy meals in thirty minutes or less so making meals from scratch is easier to fit into your schedule.

- Every weekend, plan your meals for the upcoming week and check to make sure you have the ingredients you need on hand.

- When you cook a meal, make the most of your time by preparing enough food for leftovers. You can freeze them and reheat them for dinner another day.

- Keep it simple—children prefer simple meals.

Cooking meals from scratch takes effort, but it's well worth your time. The more healthy, nutrient-dense, chemical-free foods your child eats, the better his brain and body will function.

LIMIT EXPOSURE TO PESTICIDES

The best way to limit your child's exposure to pesticides is to buy organic foods whenever possible. An organic food has been grown, handled, and processed without the use of artificial pesticides, artificial fertilizers, sewage sludge, artificial additives, hormones, or antibiotics. It doesn't contain genetically modified ingredients and hasn't undergone irradiation or been chemically ripened. In order for a product to be labeled with the *USDA Organic* seal, a government-approved certifier must inspect the farm where the food is grown to make sure that the farmer is following all the rules necessary to meet USDA organic standards. Companies that handle or process organic food before it gets to your local supermarket or restaurant must be certified as well.

The U.S. Environmental Protection Agency (EPA) has established levels of pesticide residues that are considered safe, but these levels were set based on the studied effect pesticides have on adults and don't take children into account. Children are much more vulnerable to pesticide exposure because of their smaller size and developing brain and nervous system. They may also be more sensitive to pesticides because their detoxification system is less able to adequately process and excrete them. Many people are worried because studies have linked pesticides to cancer and neurological disorders. They also disrupt **acetylcholinesterase**, a key enzyme needed for brain cell communication.

Additionally, animal research shows that certain classes of pesticides can affect the developing fetus and impair normal brain development, resulting in hyperactivity and learning and developmental disabilities. A recent research study indicated that children are primarily exposed to pesticides through their diet, and when their foods were replaced with organic foods, their levels of pesticides dropped dramatically. While you can't completely control the amount of pesticide your child is exposed to, you *can* significantly lower his exposure by purchasing USDA organic foods whenever possible.

How to Identify Organic Foods in Your Supermarket

Look for the word "organic" and a small sticker version of the *USDA Organic* seal on organic vegetables or pieces of fruit. They may also appear on the sign above the organic produce display. The word "organic" and the seal may also appear on packages of meat, cartons of milk or eggs, cheese, and other single-ingredient foods.

Foods with more than one ingredient are a little trickier. They must have at least 95 percent organic ingredients to be labeled with the *USDA Organic* seal. Food that's at least 70 percent organic can use the phrase "made with organic ingredients" and list up to three of the organic ingredients on the front of the package. If a product is less than 70 percent organic, the organic ingredients may be listed on the information panel of the package but can't say "organic" on the front. It's important to note that not all organic foods will be labeled as such because use of the seal is voluntary, so it's a good idea to read the ingredients list of every product you purchase.

Why Are Organic Foods More Expensive?

Organic foods cost more because they're produced on a smaller scale, have a lower crop yield, are subject to tighter government regulations, have high-cost farming practices, are allowed a limited number of animals per acre, and pest management is very labor intensive.

Organic foods typically cost more than non-organic foods, but prices have been coming down recently because many supermarkets have begun stocking more organic foods, and large retailers such as Whole Foods Market have become very popular. Even with the higher cost, many families are choosing to purchase organic foods for environmental and health reasons as well as to limit their exposure to pesticides.

AVOID REFINED SUGAR

Sucrose, more commonly known as white sugar or table sugar, has typically been the sugar of choice to sweeten food and beverages. Over the last several years,

high-fructose corn syrup (HFCS) has begun to replace (as well as accompany) sucrose in many processed foods in the United States. Sugar and high-fructose corn syrup can be found in soft drinks, fruit juice, candy, peanut butter, yogurt, snacks, ice cream, and many other foods our children eat on a regular basis. In fact, the average American consumes about 140 pounds of sugar each year. Think about how many empty calories that is! We all know that too much sugar is unhealthy for our children—it contributes to problems like diabetes, obesity, and tooth decay, to name a few. But does it negatively affect their behavior too? The debate over this question has been raging for decades. There are many people, particularly parents, teachers, and those in the autism community, who believe there is a definite link between sugar and behavioral problems. Parents often report that their children's behavior deteriorates after consuming foods or beverages high in sugar. In one study where primary school teachers were asked to complete a questionnaire, they overwhelmingly responded that sugar has a negative effect on students' behavior. Almost 91 percent of them also indicated that they believe sugar exacerbates behavioral problems in hyperactive children. Numerous research studies over the years support the belief that sugar has a negative impact on behavior, attention, hyperactivity, aggression, mood, and mental function. However, many other research studies conclude just the opposite, that sugar has no effect. The observations of parents and teachers that children's behavior is linked to sugar has been heavily criticized and refuted by researchers and most medical professionals.

The truth is, sugar *does* have an effect on children. Sugar is a **simple carbohydrate,** which means it is rapidly digested and broken down into glucose, which is quickly absorbed into the bloodstream. When your child consumes a sugary food or drink, it causes a rapid rise in his blood glucose level (**hyperglycemia**). This spike in your child's blood glucose level triggers his pancreas to release the hormone **insulin** to lower his blood glucose level. This in turn causes his blood glucose level to drop rapidly (**reactive hypoglycemia**), triggering the release of **adrenaline** and other hormones to raise his blood glucose level once again. Some children are more sensitive than others to this abnormal, rapid rise and fall of blood glucose levels, and their bodies overreact with a biochemical response that can lead to physical and behavioral symptoms. Symptoms vary from child to child, depending on their sensitivity, but some common ones include nervousness, shakiness, light-headedness, dizziness, fatigue, sweating, tremors, flushing, confusion, anxiety, headaches, depression, irritability, and craving sweets. The bottom line is that while sugar does not directly cause hyperactivity, it does set into motion biochemical responses in your child's body that can lead to behavioral problems.

Candy as Positive Reinforcement

Unfortunately, many therapists use candy as a reinforcer in behavioral programs or as a reward for good behavior, progress, and achieving goals. I strongly discourage this practice, and if I'm working with a child who is given candy as a reward, I ask that the therapist transition to a non-food reinforcer or reward system within two weeks. If the parents and therapist have trouble determining an appropriate reinforcer/reward system for their child, I suggest they consult with a behavior therapist. A behavior therapist can analyze your child's behavior and suggest individualized recommendations for non-food reinforcer/rewards that he will respond to. For more information or to locate a behavior therapist, visit the Behavior Analyst Certification Board (BACB) Web site at www.bacb.com.

I'm not saying that sugar is bad and should totally be avoided; instead, I encourage you to teach your child how to consume sugar responsibly to lessen its negative impact on his behavior. Your nutrition goal here is to prevent your child from experiencing hyperglycemia and reactive hypoglycemia episodes, help him maintain normal blood glucose levels, and therefore prevent symptoms such as behavioral problems. It's best to avoid high-sugar foods and drinks altogether, but that's tough to do. When your child does consume these foods, offer it along with another food containing protein. Most protein foods are also converted into glucose by the body, but this conversion takes place slowly and the glucose enters the bloodstream at a slower, more consistent rate. This will balance the effect of sugar and help your child maintain a more stable rise in his blood glucose level. Here are some more suggestions to help minimize your child's refined sugar intake:

- First and foremost, avoid high-sugar foods and beverages (anything that contains 15 grams of sugar or more "per 100 g") as much as possible.

- Replace high-sugar snacks with healthier ones such as raw vegetable sticks, fresh fruits, nuts, seeds, air-popped popcorn, fruit smoothie, yogurt, pretzels, or rice cakes with fruit spread.

- Feed your child three small meals and two to three snacks about every three hours each day.

- Make sure to provide balanced meals for your child made up of complex carbohydrates (whole grains, rice, breads, and cereals, starchy vegetables, and legumes), protein, and healthy fats.

- Offer foods that are high in soluble fiber, such as legumes, oatmeal, root vegetables, and fruit.

- Limit fruit juice to 4 ounces a day.

- Don't use candy as positive reinforcement or part of a reward system.

PROJECT NO. 1: SET THE STAGE FOR A HEALTHIER DIET

Call a Family Meeting

The first thing you should do when preparing to transition to a healthier way of eating is to have a family meeting. Gather everyone in your family together and explain *why* you're all going to start eating healthier. During your discussion, keep the focus on the entire family, *not* one particular child. (Before you call your family meeting, be sure to discuss this issue with your partner and work out any disagreements about your goals and how to reach them. It's critical that you present a united front at your family meeting.)

Clean Out Your Kitchen

Go through your kitchen cabinets and refrigerator, review the nutrition information panel on food products, and make a list of all the foods and beverages that contain artificial colors, artificial flavors, preservatives, artificial sweeteners, high-sugar, and trans fat. Gradually, over the next several weeks, replace the products on your list with healthier alternatives. Often parents are advised to immediately toss out all unhealthy foods—don't do this. It's unrealistic and may be too overwhelming a change for your family. It's much better not to toss out a food until you've purchased a healthier replacement. You're much more likely to make a successful, long-term transition to a healthier diet with this gradual approach.

Here's an at-a-glance list of ingredients you should avoid when stocking your healthier kitchen:

Artificial Colors: Artificial Color FD & C, U.S. Certified Food Color, FD & C, Blue No. 1 (brilliant blue), Blue No. 2 (indigotine), Green No. 3 (fast green), Red No. 40 (allura red), Red No. 3 (erythrosine), Yellow No. 5 (tartrazine),

Yellow No. 6 (sunset yellow)

Artificial Flavors: Monosodium glutamate, MSG, disodium inosinate, disodium guanylate

Preservatives: Butylated hydroxyanisole (BHA), Butylated hydroxytoluene (BHT)

Artificial Sweeteners: Saccharin (Sweet'N Low), sucralose (Splenda), aspartame (NutraSweet and Equal)

Refined Sugar: Sugar, corn syrup, high fructose corn syrup (HFCS)

Fat: Trans fat, partially hydrogenated oils

Now that you've eliminated foods containing chemicals and high-sugar from your child's diet and transitioned him to a healthier diet, you've likely begun to see some real improvement in his behavior, mood, hyperactivity, ability to pay attention, and overall health. (Keep in mind that your child's unique biochemical makeup will dictate how subtle or significant his behavioral changes will be.) Now it's time to move on to Step 2 —making sure your child is getting the proper amount of basic nutrients.

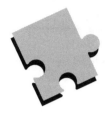

STEP 2

Make Sure Your Child Is Getting Enough Basic Nutrients

Now that you've transitioned your child to a healthier diet, it's time to focus on making sure that his diet includes enough of the basic nutrients he needs. If your child is lacking basic nutrients in his diet, his brain and immune, gastrointestinal, and detoxification systems will not function to the best of their abilities. In this chapter, you'll learn why **protein**, **carbohydrate**, **fat**, **vitamins**, **minerals**, and water are so important for your child and how to determine which of these basic nutrients he may be lacking. It's important to understand that even if your child's weight and height are within normal limits, he still may be "starving" for these basic nutrients—your child can easily consume enough calories from junk foods to gain weight and grow taller. Ensuring your child's diet includes all these nutrients is a critical part of helping him function at his best.

Unfortunately, eating a poor diet is a very common problem among children with autism. When assessing the nutritional needs of an autistic child, I ask parents to keep a food diary for three days and record everything their child eats and drinks. I've found that most autistic kids' diets look something like this: high-sugar dry cereal for breakfast, boxed macaroni and cheese for lunch, and fast-food chicken nuggets and soda for dinner. Snacks are usually junk foods, sweets, and several cups of apple juice. And of course, candy is often offered throughout the day as a positive reinforcer/reward system. It's obvious that this kind of diet is lacking the protein, calcium, fiber, omega-3 fatty acids, water, vitamins, and minerals kids need for good health.

Most American children don't eat well. Kids with autism aren't the only ones eating substandard diets. The U.S. Department of Agriculture (USDA) conducted a study on children ages two to nineteen years and found that only 1 percent of children's diets met all dietary requirements.

I know that getting your child to eat a diet that includes enough of all the basic nutrients is easier said than done. Many of the autistic kids I've worked with eat a very limited diet; some will accept only five or ten different foods. Their parents are frustrated because they've tried everything they can think of to expand their child's diet, but nothing has worked. Autistic children often refuse new foods, throw tantrums when offered a food they don't want to eat, will drink only apple juice, or seem to crave carbs. If this sounds familiar, then your child will probably not start eating a healthier diet just because you offer it to him. In Step 5, I discuss feeding problems like these in detail and offer advice on how to get your child to eat healthier foods. The information you'll learn here will focus on the basic nutrients, why they're critical for your child, and how much he should be consuming.

"When my child was diagnosed with autism, I felt hopeless. Once I moved past the initial shock and depression, I found the courage to search for answers to help my child, which started in my kitchen. I learned how to combine foods to provide proper nutrition at each meal, added healthy fats into his diet, and made sure he got basic nutrients like calcium and protein in his diet every day. Diet has become another piece of his therapy program. My son is responding well to all his therapies and moves farther from the spectrum every week."

—*Sharon, mother of a five-year-old boy on the autism spectrum*

THE BASIC NUTRIENTS

As I mentioned earlier, nutrients are divided into six categories: protein, carbohydrate, fat, vitamins, minerals, and water. These basic nutrients provide a total of forty-five essential nutrients, which our bodies are dependent on to sustain life. An essential nutrient is a substance that your body is unable to make on its own and must be consumed through your diet. Protein provides the essential amino acids histidine, isoleucine, leucine, lysine, methionine, phenylalanine, threonine, tryptophan, and valine. Fat provides the essential fatty acids linoleic acid and alpha-linolenic acid.

PROTEIN

Protein is a critically important basic nutrient, especially during infancy, childhood, and adolescence when children are growing and developing rapidly. The body uses protein to manufacture hormones, antibodies, enzymes, tissue, and neurotransmitters and to repair body cells and produce new ones. Protein can also be turned into glucose for energy required by the brain when carbohydrates are not available. Lastly, our bodies need adequate protein in order to provide **amino acids**, which are the building blocks of the body.

When your child eats a food that contains protein, his body breaks the protein into amino acids that are used throughout his body for various purposes. Some amino acids are used to produce energy during times of starvation; others are used to produce enzymes that act as catalysts for biochemical reactions and antibodies to fight off illness. Still others build muscle tissue and generate cell signaling. Several amino acids function as neurotransmitters to generate cell signaling within the brain. Some of these amino acids are involved in activities such as learning, memory, and specification of nerves in the developing brain.

If your child eats a poor diet, takes in an insufficient amount of food, or refuses to eat meats, he may have a protein deficiency. Signs of a protein deficiency include the following:

- stunted growth
- poor muscle mass
- edema

- thin and fragile hair
- decreased mental alertness, comprehension, and concentration

As you can see, protein plays a major role in both your child's body and brain function.

How Much Protein Your Child Should Eat

The chart below shows the Recommended Dietary Allowance (RDA) of protein your child should be eating based on his age. While the RDA chart will give you a good idea of the minimum amount of protein your child requires, keep in mind that he may need more protein, depending on variables such as illness, infections, stress, and genetics. It's best for a registered dietitian (RD) to assess your child's nutritional status and determine his individual protein needs and whether he's meeting them in his current diet. The RD may want to run some blood tests—for **prealbumin**, **retinol binding protein**, **transferrin**, and **serum albumin**—to assess your child's protein status. (See Appendix 1 on page 213 for more information on Registered Dietitians and how to locate one in your community.)

Recommended Daily Allowance for Protein

AGE	PROTEIN (GRAMS/DAY)	AGE	PROTEIN (GRAMS/DAY)
Children			
1–3 years	13		
4–8 years	19		
Males		*Females*	
9–13 years	34	9–13 years	34
14–18 years	52	14 years and older	46
19 years and older	56		

Source: Food and Nutrition Board, Institute of Medicine, National Academies

Choosing the Best Sources of Protein

When choosing protein-rich foods for your child, your best choices are **complete proteins**, or proteins that contain all of the essential amino acids. Complete proteins are found in foods such as:

- beef
- eggs
- milk
- poultry
- yogurt
- tofu
- fish
- cheese
- pork
- soymilk

You can also offer your child **incomplete proteins**, or proteins that lack one or more of the essential amino acids. Dietary sources of incomplete proteins include:

- beans
- seeds
- peas
- grains
- nuts

Different incomplete proteins can be combined to form a complete protein, meaning together they provide your child with all of the essential amino acids. This combination is called a **complementary protein**. An example of a complementary protein combination is beans combined with brown rice, wheat, nuts, seed, or corn; and brown rice combined with beans, wheat, nuts or seeds. See Appendix 2 for a full list of good dietary sources of protein and serving sizes.

When to Feed Your Child Protein

Many of your child's body and brain functions depend on a steady influx of amino acids throughout the day to function properly. This is especially true for the amino acids acting as neurotransmitters in his brain. Since the body is unable to store excess dietary amino acids for later use, you need to divide your child's daily protein requirement throughout the day, ideally over three meals and two snacks. Providing your child protein at every meal and snack will also help to stabilize his blood glucose levels, which will prevent hyperglycemia and reactive hypoglycemia (see Step 1 for more information on these conditions).

Many children with autism have severe feeding problems and consume a very limited variety of foods, which often results in a protein deficiency. If you're unable to increase your child's intake of high-protein foods, giving him a protein powder supplement is a good option until his diet can be expanded. There are rice, pea, soy, and whey protein supplements available that your child can use, or if he suffers from one or more food allergy or sensitivity, he could try a free amino acid–based protein supplement. As an alternative to protein supplements, you could try adding strained baby food meats to your child's foods. Baby food meats are an excellent source of high-quality protein that you can sneak into gravies, sauces, and various recipes. If you decide to give your child a protein supplement or add baby food meats to his food, you must first determine how much protein your child is getting from his current diet so you know how much more you need to add to help him reach his RDA. Then you should start with a very small amount and gradually increase the quantity each day over the span of a few weeks. Many children with autism have sensory processing disorder or sensory processing issues, which makes them very sensitive to changes in their favorite foods. These kids will reject food with even the slightest difference in flavor, odor, color, or texture. Therefore you must take the process of adding a supplement to your child's food very slowly to avoid rejection. It's a good idea to consult a registered dietitian before giving your child a protein supplement.

CARBOHYDRATE

Carbohydrates, or "carbs," are the body's primary source of energy. Proteins and fats can also serve as energy sources, but the body prefers carbohydrates because they are more easily converted to glucose. Glucose is the only source of energy the brain can use, so it's important that children take in enough carbohydrates to maintain a constant supply of glucose to the brain. This keeps their brains functioning at their optimum level throughout the day. There are two major types of carbohydrates: **simple carbohydrates** and **complex carbohydrates**.

Simple carbohydrates include monosaccharides and disaccharides. Monosaccharides, such as glucose, fructose, and galactose are composed of a single sugar unit, whereas disaccharides, such as sucrose, lactose, and maltose are composed of two sugar units. Simple carbohydrates are found in refined sugars, like the white sugar you'd see in a sugar bowl. Examples of simple carbohydrates are honey, corn syrup, high-fructose corn syrup, molasses, candy, soda, and sweets. Fruits and milk are also classified as simple carbohydrates, but they're considered nutrient-rich simple carbohydrates because they contain vitamins, minerals, fiber, and important nutrients like calcium and protein.

Complex carbohydrates are polysaccharides, which consist of many sugar units strung together to form long, complex chains. Examples of complex carbohydrates include foods such as rice, potatoes, peas, beans, corn, and whole grain products like flour, bread, and pasta. As with simple carbohydrates, some complex carbohydrates are better choices than others. *Refined* complex carbohydrates, such as white flour and white rice, have been processed, which removes nutrients and fiber. But unrefined grains still contain their original vitamins and minerals. *Unrefined* grains also are rich in fiber, which helps your child's digestive system work well.

Choosing the Right Carbohydrates for Your Child

Unrefined complex carbohydrates and nutrient-rich simple carbohydrates are far better choices than simple and refined complex carbohydrates. As I discussed in Step 1, simple carbohydrates (with the exception of fruit and milk) are digested, broken down into glucose, and enter the bloodstream rapidly, which causes hyperglycemia and reactive hypoglycemia. On the other hand, complex carbohydrates are digested, broken down into glucose, and enter the bloodstream slowly, which in turn stabilizes your child's blood glucose levels. The protein in milk and fiber in fruit prevent them from triggering the rapid fluctuation in blood glucose levels as do other simple carbohydrates.

Another helpful guide to choosing the right carbohydrates for your child is to consider their ranking on the **glycemic index**. The glycemic index ranks carbohydrates based on how they affect blood glucose levels. Carbohydrates that are digested slowly, resulting in a gradual release of glucose into the bloodstream, have a low glycemic index. Carbohydrates that are digested more quickly, resulting in a rapid release of glucose into the bloodstream, have a higher glycemic index. If your child is sensitive to fluctuations in his blood glucose levels, he may benefit from eating carbohydrates with a lower glycemic index. When he does eat a carbohydrate with a high glycemic index, he should combine it with another food that contains healthy fats, protein, or fiber to lower the glycemic index effect. The chart below categorizes common foods as low, medium, and high glycemic index for your convenience.

CLASSIFICATION	GLYCEMIC INDEX RANGE	FOODS
Low	55 or less	Whole grains, dried beans and peas, pinto beans, lentils, brown rice, popcorn, rice bran cereal, Kellogg's All Bran Fruit & Oats cereal, Special K cereal, soymilk, milk, macaroni, spaghetti, orange juice, apple juice, fruit cocktail, most fruits (except watermelon), and vegetables (except potatoes).
Medium	56–69	Wheat bread, pita bread, croissants, Life cereal, Grape-Nuts cereal, Frosted Mini-Wheat cereal, taco shell, cheese pizza, white rice, boiled white potato, sweet potato, angel food cake, macaroni and cheese, pineapple, raisins, and honey.
High	70 or more	White bread, donuts, bagels, waffle, rice cakes, cream of wheat, corn chips, pretzels, Cheerios, Corn Flakes, Golden Graham cereal, Rice Krispies, instant rice, mashed potatoes, French fries, microwave potato, instant potato, baked potato, and watermelon.

FIBER—A SPECIAL TYPE OF CARBOHYDRATE

Fiber is the indigestible portion of plants. It's considered a complex carbohydrate, but it passes through the human digestive system virtually unchanged, without being broken down into nutrients. Many children with autism have gastrointestinal problems (turn to Step 6 for an in-depth discussion on this topic), and getting an adequate amount of fiber is key to healing their gastrointestinal tracts and promoting normal daily bowel movements, which help rid their bodies of toxins. There are two types of fiber: soluble and insoluble.

Soluble fiber resists digestion and absorption in the small intestine and undergoes fermentation in the large intestine. This process results in a broad range of health benefits. For instance, short-chain fatty acids are created that promote increased proliferation of bacteria such as Bifidobacteria and Lactobacilli, which help keep the intestines healthy. In addition, soluble fiber lowers LDL (bad) cholesterol levels, helps prevent colon cancer, and keeps blood sugar levels stable by slowing the digestion of carbohydrates and the subsequent release of glucose into the blood. Soluble fiber is found in beans, peas, soybeans, psyllium seed husk, oats, barley, fruits, prune juice, and root vegetables.

Insoluble fiber absorbs water as it passes through the intestinal tract, softening stool, increasing stool bulk, and keeping things moving through the colon. Insoluble fiber is found in whole grain products, bran, nuts, seeds, vegetables, and skins of fruits.

There are three ways to figure out how much fiber your child should be consuming:

1. A study by the Child Health Center recommends that children over two years of age consume an amount of fiber that equals their age in years plus 5 grams per day (e.g., for a six-year-old child, 6 + 5 = 11 grams fiber per day).
2. The American Academy of Pediatrics recommends children eat 0.5 grams fiber per kilogram body weight. To determine your child's body weight in kilograms, divide his weight in pounds by 2.2 (e.g., for a 46-pound child, 46 ÷ 2.2 × 0.5 = 10½ grams fiber per day).
3. The Institute of Medicine has set the adequate intake of fiber at 19 grams for one to three year olds; 25 grams for four to eight year olds; 31 grams for nine- to thirteen-year-old males; 38 grams for fourteen- to fifty-year-old males; 26 grams for nine- to eighteen-year-old females; and 25 grams for nineteen- to fifty-year-old females.

I usually use the first or second method because it's a lower amount. Autistic children are already typically consuming a very small amount of dietary fiber, so I prefer to start low and gradually increase the amount of fiber in a child's diet.

Turn to Appendix 2 on page 216 for a list of high-fiber foods.

Do Autistic Children Crave Carbs?

I can't tell you how many parents I've worked with who believe their child craves or is addicted to carbs. This concept is part of something called the Opiate Excess Theory, which I discuss in detail in Step 8. It's a controversial topic, and the medical community is divided over it. Based on my years of clinical experience, I can tell you that children with autism do consume an excess amount of simple and refined complex carbohydrates. Over the years, I've analyzed hundreds of three-day food diaries, and I've seen that autistic children's diets consist mainly of the following few foods: chicken nuggets, pizza, French fries, macaroni and cheese, crackers, Goldfish crackers, cookies, pancakes, apple juice, and some fruits. With the exception of the chicken nuggets, which are a source of protein and carbohydrate, the other foods are primarily simple and refined complex carbohydrates. This preference for mainly unhealthy carbohydrates is a huge nutritional concern.

There's speculation that some children crave carbohydrates in response to the rapid brain growth that occurs during certain periods of their lives. Brain growth spurts occur between the ages of three and five, nine and eleven, and twelve and fourteen years. Interconnections within the brain increase dramatically during these times, helping the brain develop the ability to function at a higher level. During a growth spurt, there's an increase in synaptic connections between brain cells and an increase in neurotransmitter production and activity, which requires a larger-than-normal amount of glucose. As you now know, glucose is the only source of energy the brain can use, and carbohydrates are the primary source of glucose. It's possible that some children increase their intake of carbohydrates to meet this increased energy demand of their brain. Rather than limiting carbohydrates during these time periods, you should focus on providing your child with healthy, unrefined complex carbohydrates and nutrient-rich simple carbohydrates along with adequate protein.

FAT

Our bodies need fat to function properly. Besides being an energy source, fat is a nutrient used in the production of cell membranes, as well as in several hormonelike compounds called **eicosanoids**. These compounds help regulate blood pressure, heart rate, blood vessel constriction, blood clotting, and the nervous system. In addition, dietary fat carries fat-soluble vitamins—vitamins A, D, E, and K—from our food into our bodies. Fat helps maintain healthy hair and skin, protects vital organs, keeps our bodies insulated, and provides a sense of fullness after meals. It's also critical for brain function, especially in the developing brain of a child. About two-thirds of the human brain is composed of fats. The myelin sheath, which serves as a protective insulating cover for communicating **neurons** (brain cells), is composed of 70 percent fat. **Docosahexaenoic acid (DHA)** is the most abundant fat in the brain. DHA is an omega-3 essential fatty acid, which means that the body can't produce it and, therefore, must be consumed through our diet. Essential fatty acids are key building blocks of the brain and a deficiency will compromise your child's brain function, ability to learn, memory, attention, and behavior. In fact, omega-3 fatty acid deficiencies have been linked to autism, dyslexia, ADHD, dyspraxia, and depression. (See Step 4 for more information on the critical role omega-3 fatty acids play in your child's brain function.)

Types of Fat

As you can see, children need to take in a certain amount of fat for healthy brain and nervous system development. However, there are healthy fats and unhealthy fats, and it's important to make sure you're offering your child mainly healthy fats.

Healthy fats

- **Monounsaturated fat** is liquid at room temperature. Foods high in monounsaturated fat include olive, peanut, soybean, and canola oils as well as avocados, olives, and most nuts.

- **Polyunsaturated fat** is liquid at room temperature. Foods high in polyunsaturated fats include fish as well as vegetable oils such as safflower, corn, sunflower, soy, and peanut oils.

- **Omega-3 fatty acids** are polyunsaturated fats found mostly in seafood. Good sources of omega-3s include fatty, cold-water fish such as salmon, mackerel, and herring. Flaxseeds, flaxseed oil, and walnuts also contain omega-3 fatty acids, and small amounts are found in soybean and canola oils.

These fats are considered healthy because they lower LDL (bad) cholesterol and raise HDL (good) cholesterol, reducing the risk of coronary heart disease in adults. The polyunsaturated fats, particularly the omega-3 fatty acids, are especially healthy for children because they're necessary for brain development and function.

Unhealthy fats

- **Saturated fats** are usually solid at room temperature and commonly found in meat; animal products such butter, cheese, ice cream, and whole milk; separated animal fats (tallow and lard); and palm and coconut oils.
- **Trans fat** is a common ingredient in commercial baked goods such as crackers, cookies, cakes and chips, and foods fried in partially hydrogenated oils. Vegetable shortenings and some margarines also are high in trans fat.

It's fine for your child to eat foods containing saturated fats—just make sure he's eating limited amounts. Too much saturated fat can raise total cholesterol and LDL cholesterol, which increases the risk of coronary heart disease in adults. Unfortunately, many parents are told that they should eliminate fat and cholesterol from their child's diet—this is bad advice. For example, cholesterol is a major component of the myelin sheath in the brain and is critical to your child's brain development and function. The common recommendations adults are given to lower their fat and cholesterol intake are not appropriate for infants and young children. My advice is to limit saturated fat and trans fat, select more monounsaturated and polyunsaturated fats, and include omega-3 fatty acids in your child's daily diet. Your child needs fats as part of a healthy diet.

MICRONUTRIENTS

Our bodies need micronutrients, also known as vitamins and minerals, in small amounts for normal growth, function, and health. Our bodies don't make most micronutrients, so we have to get them from the food we eat or, in some cases, from dietary supplements. Vitamins and minerals are critical for brain development and function; regulating cell and tissue growth; processing and eliminating toxins from the body; maintaining a healthy gastrointestinal tract; supporting immune system function; converting protein, carbohydrate, and fat into energy; providing structure to bones; formation of blood; and numerous other body functions. Some vitamins also function as hormones, antioxidants, coenzymes, and precursors for enzymes. Each vitamin and mineral is unique and has its own specific role in the body.

The most important vitamins and minerals for brain function are calcium, iron, and some of the B vitamins:

- Calcium is required for the transmission of nerve impulses in the brain and aids in the release of neurotransmitters from neurons.
- Iron transports oxygen to the brain and is also needed to produce the neurotransmitter **dopamine**. A deficiency of iron can cause fatigue, impaired mental function, poor work and school performance, and decreased attention span, learning, and memory.
- Vitamin B_1 (thiamin) aids normal functioning of the nervous system and a deficiency can result in mental confusion and complications involving the brain.
- Vitamin B_2 (riboflavin) is required by the body for the production of energy, to form glutathione, and to convert vitamin B_6 to pyridoxal 5-phosphate.
- Vitamin B_6 (pyridoxine) helps the body break down protein and helps maintain the health of red blood cells, the nervous system, and parts of the immune system. Vitamin B_6 is also involved in the production of the neurotransmitters **serotonin** and dopamine, and a deficiency may result in depression and confusion.
- Vitamin B_{12} (cobalamin) is involved in the production of certain amino acids, maintenance of the nervous system, formation of the myelin sheath, formation of neurotransmitters, and plays a role in preventing depression and other mood disorders. A B_{12} deficiency can cause fatigue, confusion, delayed development, poor memory, depression, and neurological changes.
- Folic acid helps the body produce and maintain healthy new cells, especially during periods of rapid growth. A deficiency of folic acid may result in loss of appetite, irritability, forgetfulness, and behavioral disorders.

If your child is deficient in any vitamin or mineral, his brain won't be able to function at its optimum level. This in turn will prevent your child from fully benefiting from his various therapies and special education services. Say, for example, your child has an iron deficiency, which is a very common problem among children. As you now know, iron is essential to transport oxygen to the brain and is also involved in the production of the neurotransmitter dopamine. A low iron level could cause your child to experience symptoms such as apathy, short attention span, irritability, impaired memory, and reduced ability to learn. A recent study indicates that iron deficiency interferes with dopamine activity and may contribute to ADHD. Correcting the iron deficiency resulted in considerable improvement in these children's ADHD symptoms and cognitive test scores. If just one mineral deficiency can have such a significant impact on your child's brain function, imagine how several vitamin and mineral deficiencies can affect your child! Kids need to eat a variety of foods from all five food groups to get the basic vitamins and minerals they need for good brain and body function. However, autistic children tend to eat a very poor diet made up of only a few foods, so they often suffer from several vitamin and mineral deficiencies. If this is the case for your child, he'll likely need to take a daily multivitamin and mineral supplement until you're able to expand his diet. I discuss this topic in more detail in Step 3.

The autism community is particularly interested in vitamins B_6, B_{12}, and C because there's some evidence that they can relieve some autistic symptoms when administered at higher therapeutic levels. I cover the therapeutic use of these vitamins in steps 9 and 10.

HOW MUCH VITAMINS AND MINERALS YOUR CHILD SHOULD CONSUME

The levels of vitamins and minerals your child should consume are based on the **Dietary Reference Intake (DRI)**, which is a system of nutrition recommendations from the Food and Nutrition Board, Institute of Medicine of the National Academies. It consists of four nutrient-based reference values that were developed for different age and gender groups and are based on the average requirements for healthy individuals. Keep in mind that you should use only the DRI values as a guide because your child's actual requirements for a particular nutrient may be more or less. Here's an at-a-glance description of the four nutrient-based values:

1. The **Estimated Average Requirement (EAR)** is the average daily nutrient intake level estimated to meet the requirements of 50 percent of healthy individuals in a particular age and gender group.
2. The **Recommended Daily Allowance (RDA)** is the daily nutrient intake sufficient to meet the requirements of 97 to 98 percent of healthy individuals in a particular age and gender group.
3. The **Adequate Intake (AI)** is the daily nutrient intake estimated to be adequate for a group of healthy individuals. It's used when a RDA has not been determined yet.
4. The **Tolerable Upper Intake Level (UL)** is the highest daily nutrient intake that is likely to pose no risk of adverse health effects. It's designed to caution against excessive intake of nutrients that may be harmful in large amounts.

You probably recognize the Recommended Daily Allowance value—it's the most commonly used nutrient standard on food packages. What you need to understand about RDA values is that they're based on the assumption that your child is healthy. The RDA doesn't take into account the fact that your child may be on medications, have a chronically poor diet, or have a gastrointestinal disorder that prevents him from properly absorbing nutrients. It's also important to know that RDA values used for children are extrapolated from adult research. Some people are concerned that the RDAs don't adequately reflect the amount of nutrients kids need for optimum mental functioning. Clearly, the RDA isn't perfect, but it's the best standard currently available. When deciding how much vitamins and minerals your child should consume, I recommend that you make sure he gets at least 100 percent of the RDA. If you decide you want to give your child more than the RDA for a particular nutrient, don't exceed the UL (Tolerable Upper Intake Level). For a list of essential vitamins and minerals, their RDA or AI and UL, turn to Appendix 3 on page 222.

WATER

Water is the most basic nutrient our bodies need, and it's also one of the most neglected components of our diet. Our bodies need a certain amount of water each day for proper body temperature regulation, muscle function, absorption of nutrients, transporting nutrients into body cells, transporting waste out of body cells, and the elimination of waste and toxins from the body. We get water not only from drinking it, but also from other liquids such as milk and juice and from vegetables and fruits. If we don't have enough water in our diet, we are at risk for **dehydration**, which is a condition in which the body doesn't contain enough water to function properly. For a variety of reasons, infants and children are more prone to dehydration than adults. Symptoms of mild dehydration include the following:

- thirst
- abnormally dark urine
- decreased urine volume
- tiredness

- muscle weakness
- lightheadedness
- headache
- slightly sunken eyes

In autistic children, these symptoms can be easily missed. Autistic children often have expressive language delays or are nonverbal and unable to express their thirst. Some autistic kids don't recognize the sensation of thirst and therefore never ask for drinks. This makes them especially susceptible to dehydration. Dehydration symptoms are also often mistakenly attributed to something else. For instance, some multivitamin and mineral supplements can darken children's urine, and it may not occur to you that dehydration may be to blame instead. Subtle though the symptoms may be, dehydration will have a major impact on how your child feels both physically and mentally, his ability to function normally, and his ability to participate in and benefit from his therapy sessions.

Babies and small children have an increased chance of becoming dehydrated because

- a greater portion of their bodies is made of water;
- they have a higher metabolic rate than adults, so their bodies use more water;
- a child's kidneys don't conserve water as well as an adult's does;
- a child's immune system is not fully developed, which increases the chance of getting an illness that causes vomiting and diarrhea;
- children often refuse to drink or eat when they don't feel well;
- and they depend on their caregivers to provide them with food and fluids.

To ensure your child is both quenching his thirst and getting enough water (especially if he's nonverbal or you suspect he may not recognize the sensation of thirst), you should offer him water several times a day. If your child doesn't currently drink water or refuses it, it's probably because he's drinking too much juice or milk. Your child should be drinking two to three cups of milk and only one cup of juice a day. The rest of his fluid needs should be provided as drinking water. If your child is drinking more than one cup of juice a day right now, start cutting him back by diluting his juice 50 percent with water and gradually decrease him to one cup a day. High-sugar beverages should be eliminated from his diet altogether.

How Much Water Your Child Should Drink

The chart below lists the total amount of water your child should consume on a daily basis. When I say *total water,* I mean everything—drinking water, beverages, and water contained in foods (fruits and vegetables contain 85 to 95 percent water). The amount of total water your child needs will vary according to the level of his physical activity, medical problems, and weather environment in which you live. A registered dietitian can calculate more exactly the total amount of water your child requires based on his individual needs.

Eliminating Toxins from Your Child's Drinking Water

It's important to consider the source of the water you're giving your child, because safe, uncontaminated drinking water is vital to his health. In the autism community, neurotoxins are a major concern and many parents try to eliminate heavy metals from their

Adequate Intake (AI) of Water

	Age Group	TOTAL WATER	
		Liters/day	Cups/day
Children	1–3 years	1.3	5
	4–8 years	1.7	7
Males	9–13 years	2.4	10
	14–18 years	3.3	14
	19 years and older	3.7	15
Females	9–13 years	2.1	9
	14–18 years	2.3	10
	19 years and older	2.7	11

Source: Food and Nutrition Board, Institute of Medicine, National Academies

children's environment as much as possible. Common sources of water pollutants include the following:

- biological agents (bacteria, viruses, and parasites)
- inorganic chemicals (arsenic, lead, mercury, chromium, and nitrates)
- organic chemicals (pesticides, benzene, polychlorinated biphenyls, and trichloroethylene)
- disinfectant chemicals (chlorine, chlorine dioxide, chloramines, haloacetic acid, and trihalomethanes)
- and radionuclides (radon)

These pollutants can affect major body organs such as the kidneys and liver; promote certain forms of cancer, leukemia, and anemia; and may affect the neurological and gastrointestinal systems.

Public Tap Water

Under the authority of the Safe Drinking Water Act (SDWA), the EPA has set standards for approximately ninety contaminants in public tap water. For each of these contaminants, the EPA has set a legal limit, called a maximum contaminant level, or requires a certain treatment. Water suppliers are not allowed to provide water that doesn't

meet these standards. However, there are concerns that some of the standards for contaminants are set too high and don't protect the public against health problems. The al-
lowable amount of pesticides in our public drinking water is of particular concern
because there's been little research done on how chronic and mixed exposure to different pesticides may affect our children neurologically.

Private Well Water

Private water wells are not federally regulated, and testing of the water is the responsibility of the individual homeowner. There are numerous common contaminants found
in well water. Certain contaminants should be tested for at least once, others at least
once a year, and still others every five years, or prior to pregnancy or when an infant is
born. For information on how to test your well water, contact your state health and environmental agencies. Some state agencies and local health departments provide the
testing for free.

Home Water Purification System

Before you buy a home water purification system, I recommend that you have your water (public or well) tested by a certified laboratory. You can go to the EPA's Web site
(http://www.epa.gov/safewater/labs/index.html) or call 800-426-4791 to locate a Certified Drinking Water Laboratory in your state and find out how to go about getting
your water tested. Once you know what specific chemicals are in your water, then you
can decide whether you want to invest in a home water purification system.

There are two styles of water purification systems. A *point-of-entry* system filters all
the water you use in your home from the point at which it enters your home. A
point-of-use system is generally a filter mounted to a faucet or installed under a sink
and filters water only where it's installed. There are also many types of systems to
choose from—absorption filters, reverse osmosis, softeners, distillers, and ultraviolet,
to name a few. Whichever water purification system you choose, make sure that it's
certified by the NSF. NSF International is an independent tester of water purification systems that evaluates the manufacturer claims of reducing various contaminants and assures the consumer that the product meets performance requirements.
For more detailed information on water purification systems, visit NFS International's Web site at www.nsf.org.

Bottled Water

The major types of bottled water are mineral water, spring water, artesian water,
sparkling water, purified water, and fluoridated water. Bottled water is regulated by the

FDA and must meet EPA tap water standards; however, it's not necessarily more pure than public tap water. If you choose to drink bottled water, make sure the brand you choose is certified by NSF International. NSF has developed a voluntary certification program for bottled water, so first look for the NSF label on the bottle. If you don't see it, you can contact NSF International at www.nsf.org or 800-NSF-MARK (800-673-6275) to see if the brand you've chosen is certified or to get a list of bottled water companies that they've certified.

PUTTING IT ALL TOGETHER

The chart below serves two purposes. First, you can quickly assess whether your child is getting enough nutrients from the right variety of foods and in the proper amounts. After you've figured out what areas of your child's diet need work, you can use the chart to plan his meals and ensure he's getting the nourishment he needs. Remember, your child should be eating three meals and two to three snacks each day.

The types and amounts of food children need each day are the following:

• Milk, yogurt, and cheese, 2 to 3 servings

• Vegetables, 3 to 5 servings

• Fruit, 2 to 4 servings

• Bread, cereal, rice, and pasta, 6 servings

• Meat, poultry, fish, eggs, beans, and nuts, 2 to 3 servings

SERVING SIZE GUIDELINES FOR CHILDREN

Food Group	2–3 years	4–6 years	7–12 years
Milk			
Milk	½ cup	½–¾ cup	½–1 cup
Cheese	½ oz	½–1 oz	2 oz
Yogurt	4 oz	4–6 oz	8 oz
Vegetables			
Cooked	¼ cup	¼–½ cup	¼–½ cup
Raw	few pieces	several pieces	several pieces

(Continues)

SERVING SIZE GUIDELINES FOR CHILDREN (Continued)

Food Group	2–3 years	4–6 years	7–12 years
Fruit			
Raw	½ small	½–1 small	1 medium
Canned	⅓ cup	⅓–½ cup	½ cup
Juice	3–4 oz	4 oz	4 oz
Grains			
Bread, buns, bagels	¼–½ slice	1 slice	1 slice
Pasta, rice	¼–⅓ cup	½ cup	½ cup
Cereal, cooked	¼–⅓ cup	½ cup	½–1 cup
Cereal, dry	⅓–½ cup	1 cup	1 cup
Crackers	2–3	4–6	4–6
Meat and Dried Beans			
Meat, poultry, fish	1–2 oz	1–2 oz	2 oz
Eggs	1	1	1–2
Peanut butter	1 Tbsp	1–2 Tbsp	2 Tbsp
Beans	2–4 Tbsp	¼–½ cup	½ cup

Source: ADA Pocket Guide to Pediatric Nutrition Assessment © American Dietetic Association.
Reprinted with Permission.

PROJECT NO. 2: IDENTIFY AREAS TO IMPROVE IN YOUR CHILD'S DIET

1. *Keep a food diary, or a record of everything your child eats and drinks, for three days.*

2. *Next determine if your child is taking in enough of each basic nutrient:*

   Protein: Add up the total grams of protein your child consumed for the three days and divide by three for a daily average. Then compare your child's protein intake to his RDA.

   Is your child consuming adequate protein?

Fiber: Add up the total grams of dietary fiber your child consumed for the three days and divide by three for a daily average. Compare your child's fiber intake to his suggested intake.

Is your child consuming adequate fiber?

Water: Add up the total ounces of water (drinking water, milk, and juice) your child consumed for three days and divide by three for a daily average. Don't forget to take into account the water content of fruits and vegetables. Compare your child's total water intake to his AI.

Is your child consuming adequate water?

Fat: Did your child have at least 1 serving of a healthy unsaturated fat each day?

Variety of food groups (meat, milk, bread, fruit, and vegetables): Add up the total number of servings your child consumed from each of the food groups and divide by three for a daily average for each food group. Compare to your child's recommended number of servings.

Is he consuming an appropriate number of servings from each food group?

Did your child consume at least 1 serving from each of the food groups at each meal?

Did your child eat three meals and two to three snacks each day?

3. Choose a source of safe drinking water for your child.

Have your tap or well water tested by a Certified Drinking Water Laboratory. Based on the results, consider buying a home water purification system that can remove the contaminants in your drinking water.

The goal of Step 2 is to make sure you're offering your child a variety of foods that contain the basic nutrients he needs for his body and brain to work to the best of their ability. Once you accomplish this, you'll have successfully laid a solid foundation for all other autism therapies to build upon. Now it's time to choose a daily multivitamin and mineral supplement for your child.

STEP 3

Choose a Daily Multivitamin and Mineral Supplement for Your Child

Many healthcare professionals believe that vitamin and mineral supplements are unnecessary and that children can get everything they need just by eating a well-balanced diet. This may well be true for children who eat a variety of healthy foods, have a properly functioning digestive system that can digest and absorb the nutrients consumed, and whose bodies are able to utilize the nutrients absorbed. Unfortunately, most children with autism do not fall into this category. Children with autism often eat a very limited variety of foods. They often have mealtime behavior problems that interfere with their food consumption. Many have sensory problems that impact their acceptance of certain textures, flavors, and smells of foods, resulting in feeding problems. Some kids are on elimination diets that limit their intake of certain nutritious foods. Still other kids have chronic gastrointestinal disorders that interfere with their ability to digest and absorb nutrients properly. All of these factors make children with autism far more vulnerable to having chronic vitamin and mineral deficiencies.

Severe vitamin and mineral deficiencies, such as scurvy (a vitamin C deficiency that can result in spongy, bleeding gums, loss of teeth, nosebleeds, and, if left untreated, death), are rare in the United States. However, marginal vitamin and mineral deficiencies are very common. A marginal vitamin or mineral deficiency can result from a chronically poor diet, which impacts your child slowly, over time, with more subtle symptoms. Marginal vitamin and mineral deficiency symptoms include the following:

- poor attention and concentration
- irritability
- loss of appetite

- mood and behavior changes
- depression
- anxiety
- sleep disturbances
- susceptibility to acute illnesses such as colds and infections
- increased risk for developing degenerative diseases and cancer

Marginal deficiencies can affect your child globally, meaning they can prevent both his body and his brain from functioning at their best. Your child will be physically and mentally unable to fully respond to, participate in, and benefit from his therapies. While vitamin and mineral supplements can't replicate all the nutrients your child would get from whole foods, they're a good complement to his diet.

HOW TO SELECT A HIGH-QUALITY, OVER-THE-COUNTER VITAMIN AND MINERAL SUPPLEMENT

Vitamin and mineral supplements are a multibillion dollar industry in the United States, and there are literally thousands of products on the market to choose from with varying degrees of quality. The FDA regulates dietary supplements to some extent, but not to the same degree they do drugs. Supplement manufacturers don't need any governmental agency approval to produce and sell their products, nor does the FDA evaluate the efficacy of supplements on the market. This means that some multivitamin and mineral supplements on the market don't actually contain the ingredients or the ingredient quantity listed on the product label, may have harmful levels of contaminants, or may not break down in the digestive tract and be released into the body. Many parents get confused and overwhelmed when trying to select a supplement for their child. To simplify the task, I've listed five criteria to help you choose a high-quality daily multivitamin and mineral supplement that's right for your child.

Check Quality Control Procedures

Some supplement manufacturers voluntarily choose to have their products tested by an independent lab to verify their product's integrity, purity, and potency. Three common independent labs that test dietary supplements are the U.S. Pharmacopeia (USP), the National Sanitation Foundation International (NSF), and ConsumerLab. Each lab has its own testing standards and product verification program. The standards typically include:

- The ingredients of the supplement match what is listed on the product label.
- The supplement doesn't contain harmful levels of contaminants.
- The supplement will break down and release ingredients into the body.
- The supplement was manufactured using safe, sanitary, and well-controlled procedures.

If a supplement manufacturer chooses to participate in the verification program and passes the testing standards, they may put the verification seal on their product label. Look for the USP, NSF, or ConsumerLab seal on multivitamin and mineral supplement product labels. For more information on these independent labs, and to learn which supplement manufacturers participate in their verification programs, visit their Web sites at: www.usp.org/uspverified/dietarysupplements, www.nsf.org/business/dietarysupplements, and www.consumerlab.com/seal.

Make Sure There's a Broad Spectrum of Vitamins and Minerals

The product you choose should contain the fat-soluble vitamins A, D, and E; water-soluble vitamins B_1, B_2, B_3, B_5, B_6, B_{12}, folic acid, biotin, and vitamin C; and the minerals calcium, magnesium, zinc, selenium, manganese, chromium, and molybdenum.

You also might want to consider a calcium supplement. Vitamin and mineral supplements usually don't provide adequate amounts of calcium and other minerals. If your child is not getting enough calcium in his diet, you may need to give him a calcium supplement in addition to a daily multivitamin and mineral supplement. A calcium supplement is especially important if your child is on the Gluten Free Casein Free Diet. Research shows that autistic children's bones are thinner and less dense than the bones of children without autism. The research also indicates that autistic children on a Gluten Free Casein Free Diet have the thinnest bones of all—20 percent thinner than kids without autism.

Make Sure It Provides at Least 100 Percent of the RDA

The product you choose should contain at least 100 percent and as much as 200 to 300 percent of your child's RDA for most of the vitamins and minerals. But avoid mega-dosing at this stage. The RDA is designed to prevent a vitamin and mineral deficiency in healthy individuals and doesn't take into account that each individual has a unique biochemical makeup. It also doesn't take into consideration that your child may have a chronically poor diet, use medications, or have a gastrointestinal disorder that prevents him from properly absorbing nutrients. This means that your child may need more than 100 percent of the RDA for his brain and body to function at its best. For this reason, I typically suggest parents give their child a daily multivitamin and mineral supplement that contains at least 100 percent of the child's RDA and as much as 200 to 300 percent. Most vitamins and minerals can be increased to 200 to 300 percent of the RDA without exceeding the Tolerable Upper Intake Level (UL) (magnesium and niacin are exceptions to this rule). When using vitamins and minerals that don't have a UL determined yet, such as vitamin K and chromium, you should limit it to 100 percent of your child's RDA. At this stage, I do not recommend giving megadoses (1,000 percent the RDA) of vitamins and minerals. Megadoses of some vitamins, such as the fat-soluble vitamins (A, D, E, and K), can be potentially toxic. Vitamins A and D can cause liver damage, and vitamin B_6 can cause irreversible nerve damage. Megadoses of certain minerals can also be detrimental to your child's health. For instance, too much zinc can suppress the immune system and alter iron function. Iron can increase free radicals, intensifying cell damage, which may contribute to cancer. I recommend that you not give your child more than the UL of a vitamin or mineral without first consulting with a nutrition-oriented physician or registered dietitian. In Step 9, I discuss the use of individual nutrients such as vitamin B_6 at megadose levels, not to correct a deficiency, but to raise blood levels above normal to achieve a pharmacological effect that may improve autistic symptoms.

Avoid Certain Ingredients

The product you select should be free of artificial colors, artificial flavors, additives, herbs, unrecognized substances, and common **allergens** like wheat, milk, soy, egg, and corn.

Buy from a Reputable Company

There are many excellent high-quality multivitamin and mineral supplements on the market that do not choose to participate in the USP, NSF, or ConsumerLab verification program. Many supplement manufacturers choose to have their vitamin and mineral supplements tested by other independent laboratories to verify the quality of their products. These manufacturers have high internal standards of quality, including potency; purity in regard to heavy metals, pesticides, and other environmental contaminants; and are free of common allergens such as gluten, casein, soy, corn, and starch. Their products are also usually free of artificial colors and flavors. When researching reputable companies, your best bet is to go with a company that has a pharmaceutical background. Kirkman is a good example of a well-known reputable company that also happens to specialize in nutritional supplements formulated for children on the autism spectrum. For more information on Kirkman and the products it offers, visit its Web site www.kirkmangroup.com or call toll-free at (800) 245-8282.

CUSTOM-MADE VITAMIN AND MINERAL FORMULAS

An alternative to buying an over-the-counter multivitamin and mineral supplement is to have a vitamin and mineral formula custom-made for your child. After assessing your child, a registered dietitian or a physician prescribes the exact vitamins, minerals, and dosages he needs to function at his best. For example, if your child's immune system needs a boost, his custom formula will contain higher amounts of antioxidants. If his cognitive function needs enhancement, the dosages of B vitamins will be increased. If your child has iron deficiency anemia, iron can be added to his formula. If he's on a Gluten Free Casein Free Diet and not getting enough calcium in his diet, calcium can be added.

Customizing your child's vitamin and mineral formula has many advantages over buying an over-the-counter product. First and foremost, it's tailored to meet your child's unique needs, which is ideal. It also enables you to avoid buying multiple bottles of supplements (if your child also needs an iron and/or calcium supplement), reduces the number of supplements he needs to take each day, and simplifies his supplement program. Custom-made vitamin and mineral formulas are also superior because they

- are compounded by a pharmacist;
- are higher quality than over-the-counter formulas;
- are often covered by health insurance plans;
- can easily be adjusted as your child's needs change;
- are usually less costly than purchasing multiple supplement bottles;
- are free of allergens, unnatural fillers, binders, artificial colors, artificial flavors, and additives;
- can be naturally sweetened and flavored;
- and are available in various delivery options (liquid, powder, or capsules).

To locate a pharmacy that can compound a vitamin and mineral supplement in your area, try searching the Internet. (Using the key words "compounding pharmacy" turns up quite a few hits.) You can also contact a compounding pharmacy that I've worked with for a number of years: the Village Green Apothecary, at www.myvillagegreen.com.

GETTING YOUR CHILD TO TAKE A MULTIVITAMIN AND MINERAL SUPPLEMENT

Once you've chosen a supplement for your child, the real challenge begins—getting him to take it every day. Your child may not be able to swallow capsules yet, or refuses to eat a chewable vitamin or drink a liquid supplement. There are five different approaches that I recommend to parents I work with to get their child to take a supplement, which I describe below. Read each approach closely and then decide which one you feel will work best for your child. Be sure to start slow and be patient. Keep in mind that it won't happen overnight. It typically takes several weeks to get a child to take a supplement at the full dosage. If the approach you select doesn't work for your child, please don't give up—try another one.

Incorporate Taking the Supplement into Your Child's Behavior Therapy Program

Children with autism will often refuse a multivitamin and mineral supplement because of behavioral issues. For instance, your child may refuse to take a supplement and have a tantrum when you offer it to him. Challenging behaviors like this are addressed through various treatment approaches. Therapists often use Applied Behavior Analysis (ABA) principles and guidelines to develop an individualized behavior-based program for an autistic child. Nonfood rewards are used to help reinforce an appropriate behavior or teach a new skill. You can include taking a daily supplement without a tantrum or refusal as a new skill to be taught in your child's behavior therapy program. Rewards and strategies that are already successful with your child can be used to teach this new skill. Discuss this option with your child's behavioral specialist. Many parents I've worked with over the years have had great success with this approach.

The Pill Swallow Cup

The Oralflo pill swallow cup is a product that many parents have found very helpful in getting their child to swallow a capsule, softgel, or tablet. The pill is placed in the spout of the cup and sits above the beverage in a mesh built into the lid. Your child drinks naturally from the cup and swallows the pill and beverage together. If you choose this approach, discuss it with your child's speech-language pathologist (SLP) before starting, especially if he has any problems with oral/motor skills, swallowing, or gagging.

The Pill Swallow Program

The pill swallow program is designed to teach a child with autism how to swallow a capsule. This is not an actual "program," but a series of steps and strategies I adapted from other feeding and behavioral programs. As a registered dietitian, I don't implement this program myself. Rather I tell parents about this approach and then refer their child to a speech-language pathologist, who will actually implement and manage the pill swallow program.

Step 1: You should consult with your child's SLP to determine if he's old enough and has the oral/motor skills to safely swallow a capsule. If the SLP gives permission, then you can move forward.

Step 2: Go to your local pharmacy and buy empty pull-apart capsules in size 4. (Capsules come in sizes 4, 3, 2, 1, 0, 00; with 4 being the smallest and 00 the largest.)

Step 3: The SLP will dedicate a small portion (five to ten minutes) of her regular speech therapy session each week to the pill swallow program. Using nonfood reinforcement, the SLP will reward your child as he progresses through each step. The steps include: touch the capsule with one finger; touch the capsule with hand; pick up the capsule; place the capsule on the hand; touch the capsule to the forehead; touch the capsule to the cheek, chin, and nose; touch the capsule to the lips; tap the capsule on the teeth; touch the capsule to the tip of the tongue; lick the capsule; place the capsule on the tongue; swallow the capsule along with a beverage.

Step 4: Once your child has completed the first three steps with the size 4 capsule, repeat steps using a size 3 capsule.

Step 5: Repeat steps again using a size 2 capsule. It's usually not necessary to progress to the larger size capsules since most dietary supplements are around size 2. I've had countless parents request their child's SLP implement this program and most report back that the SLP had their child successfully swallowing capsules within a few weeks. Once your child has learned to swallow capsules, it becomes easy to administer dietary supplements as well as medications.

Negotiation

Negotiation works well with some children, especially those diagnosed with high-functioning autism, Asperger's, PDD, ADD, and ADHD. The level of cooperation you can expect from your child depends directly on his level of cognitive functioning, temperament, age, and desire to have more control over his environment. To begin the negotiation, explain to your child that he has to take a multivitamin and mineral supplement every day, why it's important, and that taking a daily supplement is not negotiable. Then tell your child that what *is* negotiable is how he chooses to take his supplement. Give him several options to choose from, such as the type of supplement (liquid, powder, or capsule) and the means by which he will take the supplement (directly by mouth or mixed in food or a beverage). If you've chosen a custom-made formula for your child, let him pick the flavor.

Mix the Supplement into a Food or Beverage

Mixing a supplement into a food or beverage is the most common approach parents try and is usually unsuccessful. Many parents are so anxious to get their child to take a vitamin and mineral supplement that they hide the full dosage in his food or beverage; he detects a difference and rejects it. Rather than starting with the full dosage, you should start with a very small dosage and gradually increase to the full dosage over the span of three to four weeks, depending on your child's sensitivity to new flavors, smells, and textures. For example, if the supplement instructions indicate your child needs 1 teaspoon of a liquid each day, the first week start with ¹⁄₁₆ teaspoon added to a food or beverage four times a day. Your child may detect a slight difference, but not enough to reject it. The second week, increase the dosage to ⅛ teaspoon four times a day. Week three, increase the dosage to ¼ teaspoon four times a day. At this point, do not increase anymore without considering your child's sensory issues and whether you think he will tolerate increasing to ⅓ teaspoon three times a day. If you go slowly, most children are able to tolerate ½ teaspoon twice a day without rejecting the food or beverage.

There are several foods and beverages into which you can mix a supplement. When considering to what food or beverage you should add the supplement, be sure it's something your child already knows and likes. This is not the time to introduce something new. Here are some examples of foods and drinks that supplements mix well with:

juice	peanut butter
milk	fruit preserves
fruit smoothie	honey
Rice Dream	ketchup
yogurt	cooked foods (after cooking)
pudding	popsicles (homemade)
juice box (inject liquid supplement into the juice box)	

Johnnie's Story

I received a telephone call from a mother recently. It was a common conversation I've had with countless parents over the years. The mother said to me, "I started Johnnie on his vitamin and mineral supplement a couple of weeks ago like you recommended. I'm seeing some improvement; he's less irritable, more focused, and sleeping better at night. Is it possible that the vitamin supplement made a difference?" My response was, "Absolutely, yes!" An observant parent will notice subtle symptom improvements when her child's marginal nutrient deficiencies are corrected with a basic vitamin and mineral supplement.

Johnnie's mother had made many attempts to give Johnnie a vitamin and mineral supplement in the past, but he always rejected it because of severe sensory issues. He refused to eat a chewable supplement. He could detect even the smallest amount of a liquid or powder supplement added to his juice or food. Out of desperation, his parents even tried crushing up a chewable tablet, mixing it in a liquid, drawing it up into a syringe, and attempted to squirt the mixture into his mouth. Of course, this method caused a huge battle and was quickly discontinued. Since it was such a challenge to get Johnnie to take a supplement, I designed a daily multivitamin and mineral supplement especially for him. The custom supplement contained 100 percent of his RDA for all vitamins and minerals, up to 300 percent of his RDA for the B vitamins, and 400 mg of calcium (the amount needed to supplement what he was already consuming in his diet to meet 100 percent of his RDA for calcium). I didn't include iron in his supplement because laboratory tests indicated his iron status was normal. The supplement was compounded by a pharmacist who added the prescribed vitamins and minerals to distilled water and sweetened it slightly with a very small amount of stevia. After the pharmacist discussed with Johnnie's mother the flavors he accepted, the pharmacist added a natural grape flavor to the liquid supplement. Johnnie's mother chose to "sneak" the liquid grape-flavored vitamin and mineral supplement into grape juice (grape juice diluted 50 percent with filtered water). She started with 1/16 of a teaspoon added to 4 ounces of grape juice. Over a period of three weeks she gradually increased the dosage of the liquid vitamin supplement to 1/8, 1/4, then to 1/2 teaspoons twice per day, which Johnnie accepted in his grape juice without a problem. Johnnie's mother was relieved that she could finally get him to take a vitamin and mineral supplement consistently every day without a struggle. She was even more amazed at how correcting Johnnie's marginal nutrient deficiencies could have such notable positive effects.

PROJECT NO. 3: CHOOSE YOUR CHILD'S MULTIVITAMIN AND MINERAL SUPPLEMENT

When deciding which multivitamin and mineral supplement is best for your child, keep in mind the five criteria:

- The quality.

- It should contain a broad spectrum of vitamins and minerals.

- It should provide at least 100 percent of your child's RDA and up to 200–300 percent without exceeding the UL.

- Avoid certain ingredients.

- Buy from a reputable company.

DETERMINE IF YOUR CHILD ALSO NEEDS A CALCIUM SUPPLEMENT

Add up the total amount of calcium your child consumed over a three-day period. Divide the number by three for a daily average and compare your child's calcium intake to his RDA. (See Appendix 3 for calcium RDA.) Is your child consuming enough calcium? If not, add more calcium to your child's diet (see Appendix 2 for sources of calcium you could add to his diet). If he still comes up short, you should add a calcium supplement to make up the difference.

Now that your child is taking a supplement every day and critical basic nutrients, vitamins, and minerals are being replenished in his body, his deficiency symptoms will begin to diminish. Your child's body and brain function will begin to improve and you can expect to see subtle improvement in his mood, behavior, and ability to participate and benefit from his therapy sessions. The next step is to increase your child's daily intake of omega-3 fatty acid.

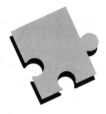

STEP 4

Increase Your Child's Omega-3 Fatty Acid Intake

As I mentioned in Step 1, essential fatty acids (EFA) are necessary fats that our bodies can't make and must be obtained through our diet. There are two groups of EFAs: omega-3 and omega-6. The levels of omega-3 and omega-6 fatty acids relative to one another are critical to the health and development of the brain and body. The optimal ratio of omega-6 to omega-3 fatty acids in our diet is four to one. Unfortunately, most American diets provide too many omega-6 and too few omega-3, the typical ratio averages twenty omega-6 to one omega-3 fatty acids. This deficiency of omega-3 fatty acids in our diet, particularly docosahexaenoic acid (DHA) and eicosapentaenoic acid (EPA) has been linked to autism, dyslexia, attention deficient hyperactivity disorder, dyspraxia, depression, and anxiety.

Research published in the April 2007 *Journal of the Developmental and Behavioral Pediatrics* supports previous research that indicates that supplementing children's diets with omega-3 fatty acids improves poor learning and behavioral problems. Another research article published in 2007 in *Biological Psychiatry* found that supplementing with omega-3 fatty acids decreased hyperactivity in children with autism spectrum disorders. Many other research studies show that supplementing with omega-3 fatty acids reduces aggression, improves reading and spelling ability, and significantly improves hyperactivity, inattention, impulsive characteristics, and anxiety as well as cognitive problems. In this chapter, we'll focus on how to increase the amount of omega-3 fatty acids your child consumes on a daily basis.

THE IMPORTANCE OF EPA AND DHA

The omega-3 fatty acids EPA and DHA play a critical role in our bodies. EPA works to increase blood flow, which influences hormones and the immune system and affects brain function. DHA is the major structural component of the brain. It supports neurotransmission among brain cells to provide optimal cognitive functioning, which impacts learning and memory. DHA is also a component of the retina of the eye, supporting optimal visual acuity (clearness of vision) and functioning, as well as vision processing. DHA is also very important during pregnancy, lactation, and infancy because of the rapid brain development of the fetus, infant, and young child. Both EPA and DHA are converted into hormone-like substances called **prostaglandins**, which help regulate cell activity and healthy cardiovascular function. Clearly, getting enough EPA and DHA is very important, especially for children.

Unfortunately, the typical child's diet is extremely low in both DHA and EPA. In fact, the average child consumes a mere 19 mg of DHA a day, which is only a fraction of the amount he should be getting. Though children do eat a small amount of the plant-derived omega-3 fatty acid **alpha-linolenic acid (ALA)**, the body must convert ALA to EPA and DHA to be useful for brain, vision, and body function. The metabolic conversion of ALA to EPA and especially to DHA is very low, even in healthy individuals.

It's also important to be aware that males are less able than females to make the conversion of ALA to EPA and DHA. Research studies indicate that children diagnosed with ADHD, dyslexia, and dyspraxia have a compromised ability to convert ALA to EPA and DHA even when they consume an adequate amount of dietary ALA. Researchers concluded that this was caused by a deficiency of the enzyme delta-6 desaturase, which plays an integral role in the conversion of ALA to EPA and DHA. It's believed that the best way to get around a possible delta-6 desaturase enzyme deficiency in your child is to provide him with a direct dietary source of EPA and DHA. That said, it's still important that your child eat foods rich in ALA because they are excellent sources of omega-3 fatty acids. The following charts list the foods that contain ALA, DHA, and EPA so you can begin to incorporate them into your child's diet.

Dietary Sources of ALA

Food	ALA (grams per 1 Tablespoon)
flaxseed oil	7.2
flaxseeds	2.4
canola oil	1.3
soybean oil	0.9
walnuts	2.6 (grams per 1 oz; 14 halves)

Source: USDA, Agricultural Research Service, Nutrient Data Laboratory

Dietary Sources of DHA and EPA

Food	DHA and EPA combined (mg per ounce)
salmon, Atlantic, farmed	608
herring, Pacific	602
herring, Atlantic	571
salmon, Atlantic, wild	521
tuna, fresh, blue fin	426
mackerel, Atlantic	341
sardines (canned in oil)	278
trout, mixed species	265
flounder	142
halibut	132
cod, Pacific	78
tuna, white (canned in oil)	69
haddock	68
catfish, wild	67
catfish, farmed	50
cod, Atlantic	45
tuna, light (canned in oil)	36

Source: USDA, Agricultural Research Service, Nutrient Data Laboratory

OTHER DIETARY SOURCES OF OMEGA-3 FATTY ACIDS

A new trend has emerged recently in which foods are fortified with omega-3 fatty acids. DHA can now be found in a variety of foods, such as infant formula, yogurt, bread, and juice. Eggs are not naturally a good source of omega-3 fatty acids, but now omega-3-enriched eggs, which contain up to 400 mg DHA and EPA, are widely available in grocery stores. Omega-3 enriched eggs are produced by feeding hens a special diet containing ground flaxseed. The actual level of DHA and EPA will vary depending on the flaxseed composition of the chicken feed. Free-range chickens that eat grass and insects also produce eggs with higher-than-normal levels of omega-3 fatty acids. Both types of eggs are good choices for your child.

"When I learned that deficiencies of omega-3 fatty acids were linked to dyslexia and attention deficient hyperactivity disorder, it caught my attention because my son Carlos is diagnosed with both these disorders. I was very anxious to add EPA and DHA into Carlos's diet, but he doesn't like to eat fish and I was also concerned about the mercury.

I tried to give Carlos cod liver oil, but he refused even the flavored ones. To add omega-3 fatty acids into Carlos's diet more naturally, I changed his milk to organic milk fortified with DHA and switched from regular eggs to the DHA-enriched eggs. I also tried Coromega, which he likes. I feel good that I'm able to provide Carlos with nutrition that is so important for his brain. I haven't seen any dramatic results, but I'm hopeful that he will gradually become more focused, less hyper, calmer, and better able to benefit from his reading therapy sessions."

—Mother of Carlos, a six-year-old child with dyslexia and ADHD

HOW MUCH OMEGA-3 FATTY ACID YOUR CHILD SHOULD CONSUME

There's no RDA for omega-3 fatty acids. Instead, the U.S. Food and Nutrition Board has set levels of Adequate Intake (AI) for ALA. No specific requirements have been set for DHA and EPA; however the Food and Nutrition Board indicates that up to 10 percent of the AI for ALA can be in the form of DHA and EPA combined. The chart below will help you determine how much your child should be consuming according to these standards.

Adequate Intake for ALA

Age of Child	ALA (grams/day)	Age of Child	ALA (grams/day)
1–3 years	0.7		
4–8 years	0.9		
Males		*Females*	
9–13 years	1.2	9–13 years	1.0
14 years and older	1.6	14 years and older	1.1

Source: Food and Nutrition Board, Institute of Medicine, National Academies

Adequate Intake for DHA and EPA (Based on 10 Percent of ALA)

Age	DHA and EPA combined (mg/day)
1–3 years	70
4–8 years	90
9–13 years	120

Source: Food and Nutrition Board, Institute of Medicine, National Academies

The National Institutes of Health recommends we consume even higher levels of DHA and EPA. According to the NIH, 30 percent of our daily calories should be DHA and EPA combined. They suggest that the intake for healthy adults be 650 mg per day. For children seven years and older who have a daily calorie intake similar to adults, the suggested intake of DHA and EPA combined is the same as adults. The chart below will help you determine how much your child should be consuming according to these standards.

Adequate Intake of DHA and EPA (Based on 30 Percent of Calories)

Age	DHA and EPA combined (mg/day)
1–3 years	390
4–6 years	540
7 years and older	650

Source: National Institutes of Health (NIH)

Since deficiencies of DHA and EPA are linked to autism, dyslexia, attention deficient hyperactivity disorder, dyspraxia, depression, and anxiety, I recommend that you follow the NIH's recommendations to determine your child's DHA and EPA needs. Here are some tips to help your child reach these levels of DHA and EPA each day:

• offer him foods rich in ALA
• purchase foods fortified with DHA
• change to omega-3 enriched eggs
• offer him a meal consisting of fatty fish once a week

Still, you may find it quite difficult to reach your child's daily goal of DHA and EPA through food alone. That's where the omega-3 fatty acid supplement comes in.

AVOIDING MERCURY CONTAMINATION IN FISH

When adding fish to your child's diet (as well as your own), it's important to consider the health concerns surrounding heavy metals like mercury and fat-soluble pollutants like PCB and dioxins. In the autism community, mercury is a heavy metal of special concern because it's a neurotoxin that harms the brain and nervous system of unborn babies and young children. Mercury naturally occurs in the environment and is also released into the air from coal-fired power plants and municipal and medical waste incinerators. The mercury travels for long distances in the air before being deposited into bodies of water such as lakes, streams, and the ocean. Bacteria in these waters transform the mercury into methylmercury. Fish absorb the methylmercury as they feed in these waters and it accumulates within them. Nearly all fish and shellfish have varying levels of methylmercury, depending on how long they live and how much other fish they eat. Basically, the larger the fish and the longer it's lived, the higher its level of mercury. When a pregnant woman eats fish, she exposes her developing fetus to methylmercury, which poses a threat to its developing brain. Depending on the level of exposure, methylmercury can cause impairment in language, attention, and memory; gait and visual disturbances; effects on neurological development; and mental retardation. The EPA estimates that 1.16 million women of childbearing age in the United States eat enough mercury-contaminated fish to pose a harmful risk to their future children.

Here are the FDA and the EPA's recommendations for choosing and eating fish for women who are or may become pregnant and nursing mothers:

- Do *not* eat shark, swordfish, king mackerel, and tilefish.

- Eat up to 12 ounces a week of a variety of fish and shellfish that are lower in mercury, such as catfish, salmon, pollock, shrimp, and canned light tuna.

- Limit canned albacore "white" tuna to 6 ounces per week due to higher mercury levels.

- Limit tuna steak to 6 ounces per week due to higher mercury levels.

- Check local advisories regarding the safety of fish caught in your local lakes, streams, rivers, and coastal areas.

- If no advisory is available, you may eat up to 6 ounces per week of fish caught from local waters, but don't consume any other fish during that week.

There are currently no recommendations regarding the amount of fish considered safe for young children, so the FDA and EPA suggest following the same above recommendations, but serve smaller portion sizes. For a complete list of fish and shellfish and their methylmercury levels, you can visit the FDA Food Safety Web site available at www.cfsan.fda.gov or call them toll-free at (888) SAFEFOOD. You can also get that information from the EPA Web site at www.epa.gov/ost/fish.

OMEGA-3 FATTY ACID SUPPLEMENTS

Since children diagnosed with autism and other developmental disorders often have sensory issues that contribute to feeding problems, eat a very limited variety of foods, and typically refuse fish, it may not be possible to get enough omega-3 fatty acids into your child's diet. If you're worried about mercury-contaminated fish, you may even choose to limit or eliminate fish from your family's diet altogether. In this case, your child needs to take an omega-3 fatty acid supplement on a daily basis.

Omega-3 fatty acid supplements are most commonly made from fish oil and are often referred to as fish oil supplements. When choosing a fish oil supplement for your child, keep the following guidelines in mind:

- Mercury and other contaminants can also appear in fish oil supplements, so be sure the supplement you choose is contaminant-free. The International Fish Oils Standards (IFOS) is the most comprehensive measurement in the fish oil industry for quality and purity. IFOS-certified fish oils are molecularly distilled in a vacuum, which results in virtually no measurable amount of contaminants.

- Look for the USP or NSF seal on the label to assure that the product has passed quality testing. You can also check the ConsumerLab Web site at www.consumerlab.com.

- As with multivitamin and mineral supplements, there are excellent high-quality fish oil supplements on the market that do not have either the USP or NSF seal on the product label. The manufacturer may choose to have its supplements tested by an outside independent laboratory to verify they're free of contaminants. If you decide to buy one of these products, be sure it's manufactured by a well-known and reputable company, like Nordic Naturals. They offer a cod liver oil product called DHA Junior that children tolerate well. It's strawberry-flavored and comes in a very small soft gel capsule, which is easy for a child to swallow or chew. Coromega is another fish oil supplement that many children accept. It's a natural orange-flavored pudding product that can be eaten directly from the packet or added to another food your child enjoys. Coromega is also great for kids because it doesn't have a fishy odor, taste, or aftertaste. For more information, visit Coromega's Web site at www.coromega.com. Both DHA Junior and Coromega are distributed by Kirkman, so you can also go to their Web site (www.kirkmangroup.com) for information on these products.

• As a general rule, naturally flavored liquid cod liver oil is a good choice for children because you need to add only a small amount and it can be easily hidden in a soft food or beverage your child eats.

Child-Friendly Fish Oil Supplements

Supplement	Serving Size	DHA and EPA (mg)
cod liver oil, flavored liquid	½ teaspoon	500
Coromega (original)	1 packet	580
DHA Junior	4 soft gels	207

TOO MUCH OF A GOOD THING?

It *is* possible to give your child too much omega-3 fatty acids. Health risks may occur if he consumes more than 3 grams (3,000 mg) of omega-3 fatty acids per day. According to the FDA's Center for Food Safety and Applied Nutrition, too much EPA and DHA may put diabetics at risk for reduced glycemic control, cause hemorrhagic stroke when taken in very large doses called "Eskimo amounts," suppress immune and inflammation responses, and cause increased bleeding if the individual is also taking aspirin or the medication Coumadin (warfarin).

You may recall from the beginning of this chapter that the levels of omega-3 and omega-6 fatty acids relative to one another are critical to the health and development of the brain and body. As you're increasing the amount of omega-3 fatty acids in your child's body, it's important that you also decrease your child's intake of foods high in omega-6 fatty acids. Foods high in omega-6 fatty acids include meats from grain-fed livestock, liquid vegetable oils (like soybean, sunflower, safflower, and corn oil), and most prepackaged and highly processed convenience foods. Consuming too much omega-6 fatty acid is associated with serious health problems, such as heart attack, stroke, arrhythmia, arthritis, osteoporosis, inflammation, mood disorders, and cancer. The omega-6 fatty acid arachidonic acid (ARA) is converted into pro-inflammatory agents called eicosanoids, which have a negative impact on the body. (Omega-3 fatty acids are also converted to eiscosanoids, but their effects are anti-inflammatory rather than pro-inflammatory.) Excess omega-6 fatty acids in our diet also compete for the same enzyme (delta-6 desaturase) needed to convert ALA to EPA and DHA, which further increases our risk for omega-3 fatty acid deficiencies. An omega-6 fatty acid deficiency is extremely rare in the United States. In fact, we tend to consume far too much omega-6 since many of us eat large quantities of grain-fed livestock and vegetable oils. As you increase the amount of omega-3 fatty acids in your child's diet, also make an effort to cut back on foods high in omega-6 fatty acids in order to achieve the ideal four to one omega-6/omega-3 ratio.

PROJECT NO. 4: INCREASE YOUR CHILD'S OMEGA-3 FATTY ACID INTAKE

1. Keep a record of everything your child eats and drinks for seven days.

2. Determine if your child is getting enough DHA and EPA by adding up the total number of milligrams (mg) of combined DHA and EPA your child consumed for the seven days and dividing by seven for a daily average. Compare your child's combined DHA and EPA intake to the recommendations by the Food and Nutrition Board or NIH on page 56. If your child is falling short, first try increasing his DHA and EPA intake through dietary sources. If that doesn't work, add an omega-3 fatty acid supplement to make up the difference.

Congratulations! Now that you've boosted your child's diet with the proper amount of omega-3 fatty acids, you've completed the first four basic steps of this program. You're ready to move into the advanced nutritional interventions. Step 5 will show you how to tackle feeding problems associated with problem eaters.

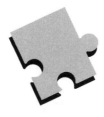

STEP 5

Resolve Your Child's Feeding Problem

Most parents of autistic children are concerned about what they perceive as their child's "pickiness" about food and negative mealtime behaviors. Autistic children tend to have poor appetites, prefer to drink rather than eat, refuse new foods, accept a very limited variety of foods, crave carbohydrates, and have a need for sameness and rituals around eating. For many families, mealtime is a battleground where their autistic child gags, throws food, or has a major tantrum, and refuses to eat. Parents try everything from forced feeding, bribing, and pleading to distracting their child during mealtime with TV and following him around the house offering bites of food throughout the day. Usually none of these techniques work, and parents are left feeling frustrated, overwhelmed, and defeated.

Unfortunately, many healthcare practitioners don't understand problem eating and negative mealtime behaviors and are unable to help parents resolve them, which only adds to the frustration. Worse yet, parents are often misinformed and told not to worry—their child will "outgrow his picky eating stage" or he'll "eat when he gets hungry enough." This is not true for kids with feeding problems, and most autistic children *do* have feeding problems as opposed to simply being picky eaters.

PICKY EATERS *VS.* PROBLEM FEEDERS

In order to help your child overcome his issues with food, you first need to determine whether he's a picky eater or a problem feeder.

Characteristics of a Picky Eater

Picky eating is a normal part of childhood development. Approximately 50 percent of children aged eighteen to twenty-three months are identified as picky eaters.

- eat fewer than thirty foods;

- eat at least one food from almost every type of food texture;

- will eat the same favorite food every day, but will eventually burn out and stop eating the food. Then they'll start eating their favorite food again after about a two-week break;

- tolerate new foods on their plate and are willing to touch or taste the food;

- and are willing to eat a new food after they've been exposed to it ten or more times.

Picky eaters tend to consume enough calories and continue to gain weight and grow without any problems. If your child is a picky eater, managing his eating is fairly easy:

- Offer your child a variety of foods each day.

- Make sure he eats his meals and snacks at approximately the same time each day.

- Create a pleasant mealtime environment for him.

- Limit his juice to 4 to 6 ounces per day.

- Limit snacks to two to three per day.

These basic strategies are usually all you need to help your picky eater eventually expand his diet to include a wider variety of foods. You can get more detailed information about managing your picky eater from a pediatric registered dietitian. Ellyn Satter, MS, RD, CICSW, BCD—an internationally recognized authority on eating and feeding—has a Web site that contains excellent information on feeding typically developing children, how to handle picky eaters, and developing healthy eating habits for your entire family. You can visit her site at www.ellynsatter.com. (Please note: If you've determined that your child doesn't have a feeding problem, you can move ahead to Step 6, Heal Your Child's Gut.)

Characteristics of Problem Feeders

Problem feeding is not a normal part of childhood development and is much more complicated than picky eating. Problem feeders tend to eat a very poor diet, may have vitamin and mineral deficiencies, consume inadequate amounts of calories and protein, and their problems may be severe enough to interfere with normal weight gain and growth. Problem feeders

- eat fewer than twenty foods;

- eat fewer foods over time until they accept only five to ten foods;

- refuse to eat foods from entire categories of texture;

- will eat the same favorite food every day, but will burn out and stop eating the food—unlike picky eaters, they won't eat the food again after a two-week break;

- won't tolerate a new food on their plate and are unwilling to even touch or taste the food;

- cry and/or throw a tantrum when offered a new food;

- have a need for sameness and rituals around mealtime;

- are very inflexible about particular foods (for example, they will eat only McDonald's French fries, not Wendy's);

- and are still unwilling to eat a new food after the typical ten exposures.

If your child has a feeding problem, he will need long-term, extensive feeding therapy from a multidisciplinary feeding team to help resolve his feeding issues.

THE CAUSES OF FEEDING PROBLEMS

Once you've determined that your child is a problem feeder, the next step is to figure out why. The only effective way to treat his feeding problem is to identify every single contributing factor to the problem. However, this is easier said than done. There are many possible causes, or combinations of causes, for your child's feeding problem, such as the following:

- medical conditions
- nutritional problems
- oral-motor dysfunction

- sensory integration dysfunction
- environmental factors
- and behavioral problems

This is where the feeding team comes in. A group of specialists—which includes a physician, registered dietitian, speech-language pathologist, occupational therapist, and behavioral specialist—will work together to identify the causes of your child's feeding problem and create an individualized treatment program to help him overcome it. A "team" is required because feeding problems are so complex, and each medical professional has a unique role to play in helping your child resolve his problem. The physician is responsible for identifying and treating any medical issues that may be contributing to his feeding problem. Each of the other therapists will conduct their own evaluation of your child to assess his feeding. Based on the results of their evaluations, the team will develop a Feeding Intervention Plan for your child. The plan will explain in detail:

- the factors contributing to your child's feeding problem,

- the strategies that will be used to address each of the contributing factors,

- specific feeding treatment approaches they will use,

- how often and with which specialist your child will have feeding therapy sessions,

- the goals for treatment and how progress will be measured,

- and how the feeding team members will communicate information to one another and to you.

As I describe the causes of feeding problems below, you'll see just how each feeding team member fits in to the process.

Medical Conditions

The first step is to have your child's physician examine him for any underlying medical conditions that could be interfering with his ability to eat. Gastrointestinal problems, such as Gastroesophageal Reflux Disease (GERD), Eosinophilic Gastrointestinal Disorders (EGID), and chronic constipation are some of the leading contributing factors to feeding problems. These conditions make eating physically painful for your child, and eventually he learns to avoid the pain by refusing to eat.

Gastroesophageal Reflux Disease is a condition where acid in the stomach backs up into the esophagus, causing it to become inflamed (**esophagitis**) and resulting in a burning sensation in the chest. GERD often occurs when the **lower esophageal sphincter** (the valve separating the esophagus and stomach) doesn't close properly, allowing acid to back up into the esophagus. Even after GERD has been identified and treated, some children still to refuse to eat because they continue to associate eating with physical pain.

Beware of Aspiration

Some children with GERD also experience **aspiration,** which is when they inhale the contents of their stomachs into their lungs. Aspiration often causes coughing and choking, but sometimes there are no symptoms. Aspiration is dangerous because it can cause infection in the lungs (like pneumonia), and it can also damage the lining of the lungs.

Eosinophilic gastrointestinal disorders are a chronic and complex group of disorders characterized by having excessive amounts of **eosinophils**, a type of white blood cell, in one or more specific places in the digestive system. For instance, if your child has **Eosinophilic Esophagitis (EE)**, he has high amounts of eosinophils in his esophagus. If he has **Eosinophilic Gastroenteritis (EG)**, his stomach and small intestines are affected; and if he has **Eosinophilic Colitis (EC)**, the problem is in his colon. The symptoms of eosinophilic gastrointestinal disorder (EGID) vary widely, depending on the area affected, and can mimic the symptoms of other diseases like inflammatory bowel disease, food allergies, irritable bowel syndrome, and GERD. (EE in particular is commonly misdiagnosed as GERD.) The most common symptoms of EGID include the following:

- nausea or vomiting
- diarrhea
- failure to thrive (poor growth or weight loss)
- abdominal or chest pain
- reflux that does not respond to usual therapy
- dysphagia (difficulty swallowing)
- food impactions (food gets stuck in the throat)
- gastroparesis (delayed emptying of the stomach)
- poor appetite
- bloating
- anemia
- blood in the stool
- malnutrition
- difficulty sleeping

If your child has EGID, it can cause him significant pain, which can result in severe feeding problems. EGID can be diagnosed only through an upper **endoscopy, colonoscopy,** and **biopsy.** Once the presence of EE, EG, and/or EC is confirmed, food allergy testing is typically ordered by the gastroenterologist. Since reactions to foods can't always be identified with food allergy testing, your child will also be put on an elimination/challenge diet to help identify problematic foods. The foods that are most likely causing your child's problem, such as cow's milk, soy, eggs, wheat, peanuts, nuts, fish, and shellfish will be eliminated from his diet first. Then they'll be reintroduced one at a time to test your child's tolerance.

Chronic constipation is typically described as infrequent, hard, and painful bowel movements. Common symptoms include abdominal cramps and pain, bloating, nausea, vomiting, irritability, behavioral problems, poor appetite, and food refusal. Chronic constipation can cause some children to develop **megacolon** (large intestines gets stretched out of shape), which causes them to pass very large bowel movements. These large bowel movements can result in **anal fissures** (tears at the anal opening), which are extremely painful. Chronic constipation can also lead to **encopresis**, or the leakage of stool. Encopresis occurs when the large intestine get stretched to the point where liquid stool leaks around the more formed stool in the colon and passes through the anus into the child's underwear. If your child has chronic constipation, the pain associated with bowel movements may cause him to refuse to go to the toilet or hold in his stool. Parents of chronically constipated kids often describe them as grazers who eat small amounts of food throughout the day rather than sitting down to eat a meal. When they do sit down to eat a meal, they tend to eat just a few bites and complain they're full.

If your child's physician suspects he has a gastrointestinal condition, he will likely refer him to a pediatric gastroenterologist for further assessment. The gastroenterologist may need to administer one or more tests to help identify your child's gastrointestinal problem, such as an **upper GI X-ray**, a **gastric-emptying study**, an **upper GI endoscopy,** or a **pH probe**.

It's also important that your child be seen by a registered dietitian. She can assess whether there are dietary factors contributing to his gastrointestinal problems, such as lack of fluid and fiber intake, medication effects, problematic foods, excess juice intake, and nutrient deficiencies. (Turn to Step 6 for a more in-depth look at gastrointestinal problems in children on the autism spectrum.)

Food Allergies, Sensitivities, and Intolerances

If your child suffers from a food allergy, sensitivity, or intolerance, it may cause him to have several intestinal symptoms, such as reflux, nausea, vomiting, abdominal pain, abdominal distension, gaseousness, loose stools, diarrhea, and chronic constipation. Naturally, these symptoms will make your child feel very uncomfortable, and he'll learn that eating makes him feel bad. Your child may often refuse food, gradually limit the number of foods he's willing to eat, and have tantrums and behavioral problems at mealtime. Be sure to rule out food allergies, sensitivities, and intolerances as a possible contributing factor to your child's feeding problem. (Step 7 discusses in detail how you can identify a problematic food and the appropriate nutritional treatment.)

Medication Side Effects

Many children with autism and related disorders take medication to treat issues like depression, obsessive compulsivity, aggression, tantrums, hyperactivity, and attention deficient. The most common medications used are antidepressants (Anafranil, Luvox, Prozac, Paxil, Zoloft, Lexapro), antipsychotics (Clozaril, Risperdal, Zyprexa), and stimulants (Ritalin, Adderall, Dexedrine). These medications can cause side effects that contribute to a feeding problem. Common side effects include the following:

- decreased or increased appetite
- decreased or increased weight
- nausea
- vomiting
- dry mouth

- altered taste
- abdominal pain
- loose stools
- diarrhea
- constipation

Your child may also have other conditions that are being treated with medication, such as a sleep disorder, seizures, allergies, or digestive problems. If your child is taking one or more medications, you should have a registered dietitian review the potential side effects and assess whether they're contributing to his feeding problem. Keep in mind that your child should never stop taking a prescribed medication without first discussing it with his physician.

Previous Invasive Interventions

Some children who've had an invasive procedure performed around the mouth, such as intubation, tracheostomy, or a nasogastric feeding tube, have ongoing feeding problems for months, and even years, after the tubes have been removed. This can happen when a child is physically unable to eat for an extended period of time and misses the critical developmental stage necessary to build a foundation for feeding skills and normal eating behaviors. It can also occur when a child is traumatized by an invasive procedure and develops a fear of putting things, including food, into his mouth.

Dental Problems

Dental issues such as **caries**, sore or swollen gums, and mouth sores can contribute to a feeding problem. Your child may limit his diet to soft, smooth foods and refuse crunchy, spicy, or hot foods. Have his dentist rule out dental issues, and be sure your child is going for regular check-ups and cleanings.

Nutritional Problems

Nutritional problems are a common but often overlooked contributing factor to feeding problems. Many times, these problems can be relatively easy to fix. For instance, if your child is drinking too much juice, it can fill up his stomach and make him feel full at mealtimes, preventing him from eating solid foods. Children should have only 4 to 6 ounces of juice per day, but many children drink much more than that. I know kids who sip juice throughout the day and take in as much as 32 to 48 ounces per day. If your child is drinking an excess amount of juice, you should gradually decrease the total amount to no more than one cup per day. You may find that this not only improves your child's appetite but also his loose stools.

Nutrient Deficiencies

You may remember from Step 3 that a common symptom of vitamin and mineral deficiencies is loss of appetite. This is particularly true of a zinc deficiency. Deficiencies of other vitamins and minerals can have global symptoms, such as irritability, mood and behavior changes, decreased attention, and lethargy, which can interfere with your child's ability to sit down at the table and eat a well-balanced meal. It's a vicious cycle: A poor diet causes nutrient deficiencies, which in turn leads to poor appetite, which results in food refusal and mealtime behavior problems. Turn to Step 3 for a refresher on improving your child's diet with a daily multivitamin and mineral supplement. A registered dietitian can assess your child's diet to determine specific vitamin and mineral deficiencies and recommend appropriate supplements.

Oral-Motor Dysfunction

Your child may have an oral-motor skill problem, such as difficulty sucking, biting, chewing, swallowing, or coordinating tongue movements, which interferes with his ability to eat and to handle foods of certain textures and consistencies. A speech and language pathologist (SLP) can evaluate your child's oral-motor function, identify delays and problems, and then guide him through therapeutic activities that will improve his feeding skills. The SLP may have your child undergo an X-ray procedure called a **video fluoroscopic swallow study** (also known as a **modified barium swallow study**) to determine whether he's able to swallow safely without aspirating food or liquid into his lungs. It's very important that your child be assessed by a SLP before starting a feeding therapy program. This serves two purposes: You'll be able to rule out or identify and treat any oral-motor problems, and you'll also reduce your child's risk for aspiration and choking.

Sensory Integration Dysfunction

One of the leading contributors to feeding problems among autistic children is **sensory integration dysfunction**, also known as sensory processing disorder. Children with sensory integration dysfunction experience a disruption of the intake and organization of sensory information within the brain. This causes them to have trouble responding appropriately to sensory information from their environment. Sensory processing dysfunction affects children in every facet of their lives, including eating. Eating is a complex act that requires all five of our senses: visual, tactile (touch), smell, taste, and auditory (hearing). Your child must be able to simultaneously integrate all five of his senses during the eating process. If he has sensory integration dysfunction, he likely has a tough time touching, let alone eating, food. He may be hypersensitive to the texture, smell, and temperature of foods and become easily overwhelmed during mealtime, triggering a tantrum and food refusal. Your child may also overreact to noises and be unable to eat at mealtime when family members are talking at the dinner table. Conversely, your child may be hyposensitive and is not sensitive *enough* to sensory information. This would prompt him to seek out constant stimulation or more intense sensory experiences. Hyposensitive children often stuff their mouths full of food, pocket food in the sides of their mouths, and swallow the food later or spit it out.

Here are some common mealtime responses you may have seen from your child if he has sensory issues:

Visual. Your child may prefer foods of a certain color and reject foods of any other color. He may have a tantrum if foods touch each other on his plate. Serving sizes that are too large may visually overwhelm your child and he may totally refuse to eat anything.

Tactile. If your child is hypersensitive, he may be unwilling to touch foods with his hands. (Exploring foods with his hands is a critical step to becoming familiar with a new food, putting it in his mouth, and learning to successfully eat it.) He likely rejects new foods, and gags, chokes, or vomits, which reinforces his fear of certain foods.

Smell. If your child is hypersensitive to smells, he may become fussy and eventually totally overwhelmed by the odors of food preparation and cooking before mealtime even begins. He may gag or vomit when the food is offered at mealtime.

Taste. Strong flavors can trigger the gag reflex in children with taste hypersensitivity. Your child may have very strong taste preferences and prefer bland foods or specific flavors.

Auditory. For children who are hypersensitive to sound, eating food itself can create sounds that are overwhelming. Your child may prefer soft foods and liquids to avoid the sounds created by hard, crunchy foods. People talking at the table, sounds in the environment, television, and other sounds during mealtime may distract your child and he may be unable to eat.

If your child is hyposensitive to sensory input, he may seem oblivious during mealtimes, even in noisy environments. He may have trouble differentiating between different tastes, textures, temperatures, and smells of food. He may also have trouble identifying when he's full, which can lead to portion control issues.

An occupational therapist (OT) can evaluate your child's ability to process sensory information, assess if he has a sensory integration dysfunction, and identify how it impacts his ability to eat. The OT plays a major role in developing a feeding therapy program, providing therapy, and improving your child's tolerance level to sensory input.

Environmental Factors
Your child's mealtime environment plays an important role in his ability to eat.

Distractions. Distractions during mealtime can over-stimulate your child; he may become overwhelmed from the sensory overload, lose focus, and lose interest in eating. Be sure to keep distractions at mealtime to a minimum by limiting noise and turning off the television set.

Grazing. If your child picks at food all day long and never sits down for a real meal, he'll lose his internal biorhythm of feeling hungry and full. He won't develop normal hunger cues and won't have the desire to sit down and eat a meal or healthy snack.

Lack of routine. Children should have a structured schedule that includes three meals and two to three snacks every day. Otherwise, they can't fall into a comfortable pattern of expecting meals and snacks. Offer your child his meals and snacks at a designated place where he's expected to sit in a chair at a table. Consistency, structure, and routine developed around meals and snacks will promote a healthy appetite and improved eating.

Mealtime dynamics. Your interaction with your child at mealtime may also play a role in his feeding problem. For instance, trying to coerce, trick, or bribe your child to taste a food will lead to struggles between you that will only worsen his problem.

Improper physical environment. Where your child sits, his chair, his posture during mealtime, and the utensils he uses all need to be assessed to make sure they meet his needs. For instance, your child's utensils may not be age-appropriate. Or he may need a more supportive chair to facilitate eating.

I encourage you to have one of your child's therapists and/or a behavioral therapist come to your home and observe a mealtime. This is the best way to identify any environment factors that need to be addressed and come up with strategies to resolve them that can be included in your child's feeding therapy.

Behavioral Problems

Your child's behavior toward food and at mealtimes is the final piece in the feeding problem puzzle. It's very important to pay attention to your child's negative mealtime behaviors because he's trying to tell you something. If you learn to interpret his behaviors, you'll be able to figure out where the feeding process is breaking down for him. Common negative mealtime behaviors include the following:

- refusing to come to the table
- not sitting still in his chair and continually leaving the table
- refusing to eat
- throwing food
- crying when presented with food
- throwing tantrums
- gagging and/or vomiting
- spitting out food
- disrupting others who are trying to eat

As you now know, many of these behaviors could be caused by medical conditions, nutritional problems, oral-motor dysfunction, sensory integration dysfunction, and environmental factors. Once all of the issues I've discussed in this chapter have been ruled out or identified and addressed in your child's treatment program, you may find that his behaviors at mealtime improve significantly. However, these negative responses may be so entrenched in your child's mealtime routine that he continues them even after the root problem has been resolved. I strongly recommend that you have your child assessed by a behavioral specialist. The behavioral specialist will conduct a behavioral functional assessment, which will help determine what triggers specific behaviors at mealtime, and develop strategies for you to handle your child's behavior. He can also advise the other therapists on your child's feeding team on how to best handle your child's behavior problems and offer insight on his feeding intervention plan.

Tyler's Story

Tyler was a twenty-seven-month-old diagnosed with PDD-NOS. He was also a twin who had been born two months premature. His parents told me he was nonverbal, avoided contact with other people, had severe "meltdowns," and often spun around in circles. He had been receiving speech therapy once a week through an Early Intervention program and had an Individual Family Service Plan (IFSP) in place.

Tyler's parents described him as a very picky eater. In reality, Tyler had a severe feeding problem. He only ate Stage 2 baby foods (sweet potato, pears, and vegetable/chicken), chocolate-flavored soy milk, water, and GFCF potato chips, and had never transitioned to regular table foods. He once tried to eat shredded chicken but spit it out after he chewed it. Tyler did not express hunger, refused to try new foods, refused baby foods he used to eat, and resisted going to the table at mealtime. On the other hand, Tyler's twin brother had transitioned to regular table foods without a problem and was eating a wide variety of foods. In an attempt to get Tyler to eat, he was allowed to "graze" on foods and sip chocolate-flavored soy milk from a sippy cup all day long. His mother said that the only way she could get Tyler to eat at all was to sit him in front of the television and distract him during mealtime. His parents were very frustrated and simply didn't know what else to do. Tyler was not receiving any type of therapy to address his feeding problem.

To start, I sent a letter to Tyler's physician explaining that I suspected Tyler was not a picky eater, but rather he had a severe feeding problem that required an evaluation and feeding therapy by a multidisciplinary feeding team. Tyler was then referred to a pediatric gastroenterologist to rule out any medical conditions that may be contributing to his feeding problem, especially since as an infant he had a history of reflux, projectile vomiting, and required an amino acid–based infant formula. Tyler was also evaluated by the occupational therapist with the early intervention program to determine if his sensory integration processes were impacting his feeding. His speech language pathologist expanded on her speech evaluation to assess his oral-motor and swallow skills related to feeding. I also suggested a referral to a behavioral specialist who could evaluate Tyler's behavior and interactions with his parents during mealtime.

Following my recommendation, Tyler's mother requested an IFSP meeting, where she asked that feeding therapy be included in Tyler's IFSP. It was designated that the speech language pathologist would provide two feeding therapy sessions a week. The speech language pathologist wanted to do this, but didn't feel she had adequate training in the area of feeding therapy. After additional negotiation, the early intervention program agreed to send the speech language pathologist to Dr. Toomey's two-day seminar to learn the SOS approach to feeding. She returned from the intense comprehensive training prepared and excited to get started with Tyler. Together, the entire feeding team—Tyler's parents, the speech language pathologist, occupational therapist, behavioral specialist, and the registered dietitian—developed a feeding intervention plan and wrote feeding outcomes and objectives that were included in Tyler's IFSP. Tyler began his twice weekly feeding sessions and within just eight weeks, significant improvements were made. Tyler accepted six solid foods: GFCF cookies, crackers, and bread, rice cakes, peanut butter, and bacon. After several more weeks, his diet expanded even more to include vegetables, fruit, and meat. With the entire feeding team working together, Tyler accomplished the goal of eating a developmentally age-appropriate meal, sitting in a chair at the table, and using age-appropriate utensils to feed himself.

Tyler's mother did an outstanding job of pulling together a feeding team with the cooperation of the Early Intervention program. She strongly and successfully advocated for her son and received services that were not traditionally provided by that particular program. Tyler's mom told me that it was a very hard task to accomplish and extremely frustrating at times, but she was determined not to give up. She said, "Every minute was worth it when my husband and I can sit down at the dinner table and enjoy a normal meal with both our boys."

INDEPENDENT FEEDING THERAPY PROGRAMS

There's very little research available on effective therapy to treat feeding problems among young children with autism, and even less information on working with older children. However, there are a few step-by-step feeding therapy programs that have been quite successful with autistic children. Cheri Fraker, CCC-SLP, has created a program called Food Chaining, which is based on the idea that there are specific reasons why your child will eat only certain foods. Your child may find these foods acceptable because of their color, texture, flavor, or even visual appearance. Food chaining determines why your child accepts certain foods, and then shows you how to expand his food repertoire by introducing new foods that have the same features as the ones he currently eats. After your child has expanded his diet with this method, new foods with slightly different features are introduced. You can find a complete description of this method in *Food Chaining: The Proven 6-Step Plan to Stop Picky Eating, Solve Feeding Problems, and Expand Your Child's Diet,* by Cheri Fraker, Laura Walbert, Sibyl Cox, and Mark Fishbein.

Another feeding therapy program that has proven effective is the Sequential Oral Sensory (SOS) Approach to Feeding, which was developed by pediatric psychologist Dr. Kay Toomey. The SOS approach is a thirty-two-step plan designed to ease your child into tolerating, interacting, smelling, touching, tasting, and eating a new food. Dr. Toomey offers advanced courses to train therapists in the SOS approach in Denver, Colorado.

If you're considering trying either one of these treatment approaches, be sure to discuss it with your child's feeding team first.

FINDING A FEEDING TEAM

Many hospitals, medical facilities, and private clinics in large cities have feeding teams already in place. However, if you don't live in or near a large city, this may not be a good option for you. Feeding therapy is intensive and can last for months, and it's unrealistic for you to drive back and forth long distances for feeding therapy sessions for an extended period of time. If you live in a smaller town or a rural area, chances are you won't find an already-assembled feeding team in your community. This means you're going to have to put one together on your own. Before you panic at the thought, let me assure you that assembling a feeding team for your child is not as hard as you might think. The following steps will help you get started:

1. Start by looking at the therapists who are already treating your child's autism. Do any of them have experience with feeding problems? If so, talk to them about becoming part of your child's feeding team.

2. Ask your child's physician for referrals to a speech-language pathologist, occupational therapist, registered dietitian, and behavioral specialist.

3. Set up a time to talk with each of the referrals. You want to get to know them a bit, as it's important for you and your child to feel comfortable with everyone on the feeding team, and you should also find out if they have experience with autism and feeding problems.

4. Once you have selected the members of your child's feeding team, schedule an appointment with each of the therapists for a comprehensive assessment.

5. Ask the feeding team to develop a Feeding Intervention Plan for your child.

Putting together your child's feeding team will take some work, but it's the only way you're going to be able to resolve his feeding problem and expand his diet. In the end, I know you'll find that it's well worth the effort.

AT-HOME STRATEGIES TO IMPROVE YOUR CHILD'S FEEDING PROBLEM

It's going to take some time to locate or assemble a feeding team, have your child evaluated, develop a feeding intervention plan, and start feeding therapy sessions. In the meantime, here are some very basic strategies you can use to improve your child's feeding problem.

Use positive reinforcement. Praise your child when he does something appropriate at mealtime, and do your best to ignore his negative behaviors. Do the same with your child's siblings to help reinforce the point. Keep mealtime positive, pleasant, and enjoyable.

Use social modeling. Even if your child refuses to eat, have him sit at the dinner table with the rest of the family at mealtime. You and your child's siblings should model good eating and social behavior and avoid making negative comments and faces at foods. Your child should not be the focus of the mealtime.

Limit his juice. Don't allow your child to drink more than one cup of juice per day.

Don't let him graze. Your child shouldn't be nibbling on small amounts of food all day long. Offer him three meals and two to three small snacks per day. Offer him water between meals and snacks.

Stick to a schedule. Your child's meals and snacks should be approximately two and a half to three hours apart and offered at approximately the same time and at the same place in your home every day. He needs to learn that there's a consistent daily routine for meals and snacks. Meals should be limited to no more than thirty minutes and snacks to fifteen minutes.

Limit distractions during mealtime. Turn off the television during meals, and keep the ambient noise level down to avoid auditory over-stimulation.

Offer manageable foods. Present foods on your child's plate in small, easily chewable bites. There should be no more than three different foods on his plate at any one time. Give your child smaller-than-normal serving sizes to avoid visual over-stimulation.

Get your child involved. Make your child a part of menu planning, grocery shopping, food preparation, and setting the table for meals. He's more likely to eat a food if he's had some sort of interaction with it prior to mealtime.

Use appropriate mealtime language. Don't ask your child a question or make a demand to which he can respond with a "no." This will lead to a power struggle between you. Avoid "can you?" questions and "don't" demands. Instead, speak to your child using positive statements, such as "you can" and "do." Here are some examples:

Instead of saying "Suzie, can you take a bite of peas for Momma?" say, "Suzie eats peas with her spoon."

Instead of saying "Suzie, please can you drink some milk for Daddy?" say, "Suzie sips milk from her cup."

Instead of saying "Don't throw your cup!" say, "Cups are for drinking. Your cup goes here until you're ready to take a sip."

Instead of saying "Don't put so many crackers in your mouth at a time! You're going to choke!" say, "Johnnie chews one cracker at a time."

Avoid food burnout. If your child eats the same food, the same way, every day, he'll eventually "burn out" and eliminate the food from his diet. Once an autistic child with a feeding problem eliminates a preferred food, he usually won't accept it again in the future. If your child continues to burn out on his preferred foods, he'll soon be left with a very few foods in his diet. To avoid burnout, offer a particular food no more than every other day; and if your child has a very limited food repertoire, and you have no choice but to offer a particular food daily, change one thing about the color, shape, texture, or taste of the food. The change should be very slight—your child should notice a difference but not enough to cause him to reject the food. Even a difference this slight can be enough to prevent food burnout. Here's an example:

Suzie eats a pancake every day, but her diet is limited to three foods, so her mom has to offer them every day and avoid burnout at the same time.

Monday: Mom should serve the pancake as usual.

Tuesday: Mom should change the shape; for instance, make it oblong instead of perfectly round.

Wednesday: Mom should change the taste; for instance, add two eggs to the batter instead of one.

Thursday: Mom should change the texture; for instance, add a very small amount of fiber powder to the batter.

Friday: Mom should change the color; for instance, add a small amount of fruit preserve to the batter.

Saturday: Mom should change the shape of the butter on the pancake.

Sunday: Mom should change the color of the syrup; for instance, make it darker or lighter.

These basic strategies will help you get started improving your child's eating behaviors and hopefully prevent them from getting worse while you wait for his feeding therapy to begin.

PROJECT NO. 5: DETERMINE WHETHER YOUR CHILD IS A PICKY EATER OR A PROBLEM FEEDER

1. Consult the list of characteristics for picky eaters and problem feeders on pages 61–63. If your child demonstrates characteristics of a picky eater, see a registered dietitian for strategies to handle picking eating.

2. If your child demonstrates characteristics of a problem feeder, take him to his physician for a complete medical exam and ask if he can refer you to a feeding team.

3. If your child's physician can't refer you to a feeding team, assemble the team yourself by consulting with your child's current therapists and/or getting individual referrals from your child's physician (see page 74 for tips on putting together a feeding team on your own).

4. Start implementing the at-home feeding strategies to help improve your child's feeding.

My hope is that you come away from this chapter with an understanding of how important it is to address and resolve your child's feeding problem. You can't take a "wait and see" approach and hope your child's feeding problem improves on its own. It won't. In fact, it will only worsen over time. The sooner you take action, the better. It's also important to recognize that you *cannot* solve your child's feeding problem on your own. Feeding problems are very complex, and your child must be treated by a team of professionals. It's true that Step 5 is time-consuming, and it will take weeks or even months to achieve. But watching your child's diet expand, and seeing him eat a variety of healthy foods, probably for the very first time, is a wonderful reward for all your time, effort, and hard work.

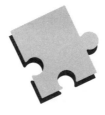

STEP 6

Heal Your Child's Gut

Gastrointestinal problems involving the esophagus, stomach, small intestine, and colon are very common among children with autism. In fact, recent research shows that GI problems are more prevalent in autistic kids than other children, a notion that the medical community had long dismissed as improbable. In a study published in the *Journal of the Developmental and Behavioral Pediatrics* in 2006, 70 percent of autistic children were found to have a lifetime history of gastrointestinal symptoms such as abnormal stools, constipation, frequent vomiting, and abdominal pain. Other research studies indicate that children with autism have high rates of **lymphonodular hyperplasia (LNH)**, **esophagitis**, **gastritis**, **duodenitis**, and **colitis** as well as low levels of intestinal carbohydrate digestive enzymes. The symptoms of gastrointestinal problems, which range from mild to severe, can have a major impact on both your child's health and his behavior. If your child suffers from one or more of the symptoms listed below, a gastrointestinal disorder may be the culprit:

- abdominal pain
- constipation
- vomiting
- bloating
- reflux
- diarrhea
- gaseousness

If your child is indeed suffering from a gastrointestinal disorder, effective treatment will resolve his symptoms, which in turn should improve some of his behaviors.

We don't know exactly why such a large percentage of autistic children suffer from gastrointestinal disorders, but there are countless theories. Some believe that autistic children suffer from **leaky gut syndrome** (increased intestinal permeability); others think that it's due to an imbalance of microflora in the gastrointestinal tract (specifically, the overgrowth of *Candida albican* yeast). Some believe an autoimmune disease is to blame, and still others think it's caused by IgG food sensitivities or carbohydrate digestive enzyme deficiencies. There's also talk about a new variant form of inflammatory bowel disease called **autistic entercolitis**, which was first reported by gastroenterologist Dr. Andrew Wakefield and is very controversial. In the end, it doesn't really matter *why* your child is more prone to GI problems; what matters is identifying and healing the problem.

ELIMINATION PROBLEMS

The most common complaints children with autism seem to have when it comes to GI problems is chronic constipation, chronic diarrhea, and loose or nonformed stools. Research confirms that constipation is more common in children with autism than other children. Abdominal X-rays of children with and without autism who are experiencing stomach pain have shown that autistic children have a significantly higher rate of excess stool in the colon. Children with chronic constipation often associate bowel movements with pain and deliberately hold in their stool to avoid a bowel movement. Holding in their stool causes them to lose the urge to have a bowel movement, which completes the vicious cycle that is chronic constipation. If your child is experiencing chronic constipation, he's at the very least uncomfortable and may well be in pain. As you may remember from my discussion of chronic constipation in Step 5 (see page 66), it can result in physical issues such as megacolon and encopresis and behavioral issues that contribute to feeding problems.

To help you assess whether your child may be constipated, the chart below shows the average number of bowel movements you should expect from your child throughout his childhood years. If he's falling short within his age group, talk to his physician.

Age	Number of Bowel Movements	
	per Day	*per Week*
0–3 months		
breastfed	2.9	5–40
formula fed	2.0	5–28
6–12 months	1.8	5–28
1–3 years	1.4	4–21
Over 3 years	1.0	3–14

Source: ACTA Paediatrica Scandinavica (Stockholm) 1989; 78:682-4

On the other end of the spectrum, autistic children also tend to have problems with chronic diarrhea, loose stools, nonformed stools, or a combination of all three at different times. Many parents describe their child as never having had a normally formed stool. Chronic diarrhea is diarrhea that's present for more than three weeks and is not associated with an illness. Many medical professionals refer to it as chronic nonspecific diarrhea (CNSD). If a child with CNSD continues to gain weight and grow taller at a normal rate, many medical professionals don't consider it a significant health problem or suggest any specific medical treatment to resolve the issue. Parents, however, are usually very concerned about their child's abnormal stools and rightly so. If your child is having difficulty controlling his bowel function, it will impact him in many ways. For instance, having chronic diarrhea, loose stools, and/or nonformed stools will affect his ability to potty train, forcing you and other caregivers to continue changing diapers beyond the typical age. Your child's bowel function issues may make him feel uncomfortable and self-conscious, which will affect his sensory system and can lead to behavioral problems. He may also encounter nutritional deficiencies because chronic diarrhea causes malabsorption of vitamins, minerals, omega-3 fatty acids, and other nutrients. This impedes his body's ability to repair the lining of the GI tract, which serves only to exacerbate his malabsorption of nutrients. This vicious cycle of chronic diarrhea, malabsorption, and nutrient deficiencies can compromise your child's overall health, brain function, and behavior.

THE GI DISORDER—BEHAVIOR CONNECTION

Undiagnosed GI disorders can cause serious behavioral problems in autistic children, particularly those who are unable to verbally express the pain they're feeling. If your child is nonverbal, the only way he can communicate how he feels is through his behavior. Some common behaviors that may indicate your child has a GI disorder are the following:

- food refusal
- accepting a limited variety of foods
- mealtime tantrums
- irritability
- self abuse

Unfortunately, too often these symptoms are dismissed "typical" autistic behaviors as opposed to attempts to communicate what can't be put into words. Identifying and correcting your child's GI disorder will lead to significant improvement in the way he behaves.

Sara's Story

Eight-year-old Sara was diagnosed with autism; she was nonverbal and had severe behavioral problems, including self abuse. Sara's mother informed her speech and language therapist that Sara was a picky eater (she was really a problem eater as she ate only three foods) and had severe behavioral problems at mealtime, such as throwing food, crying, tantrums, and biting herself. Since Sara was nonverbal, the first thing the SLP did in speech therapy was to teach Sara to use colors as a way to express herself. Each color represented a feeling; for example, the color red meant mad, angry, pain, or hurt. After Sara learned the colors, the SLP encouraged her to draw a picture. Sara took a crayon and drew a stick figure of a person. Then she picked up the red crayon and drew a red ball in the stomach area and a red line up to the center of the chest area of the stick figure. The SLP shared the picture with Sara's parents, who took her to a pediatric gastroenterologist. The GI specialist performed several studies, including an upper GI endoscopy, and discovered Sara was suffering from GERD with severe esophagitis. Sara had probably been suffering from undiagnosed GERD and esophagitis for years, experiencing severe pain after mealtime but unable to verbally express how she felt. Sara's behavior at mealtime was her way of communicating her pain, but instead everyone thought she was merely having typical autistic behavioral problems.

CONTRIBUTING FACTORS

The factors that contribute to gastrointestinal problems can be split into two categories: dietary and physical. If your child is expressing one or more of the GI symptoms listed on page 79, you need to figure out what specific factors are contributing to his symptoms. Then you'll be able to determine the medical and dietary treatments that are right for him. Common contributing factors include the following:

- inadequate water intake
- inadequate dietary fiber intake
- low muscle tone (**hypotonia**) or increased muscle tone (**hypertonia**)
- decreased physical activity
- irregular toilet habits
- unable to communicate the need to have a bowel movement

- holding in his stool
- medication side effects
- excessive or long-term use of laxatives, suppositories, and enemas
- malnutrition
- cow's milk allergy
- medical conditions

DIETARY TREATMENT

The first thing you should do is adjust your child's diet. Making specific dietary modifications, adding basic and advanced supplements to his diet, and identifying and eliminating problematic foods can vastly improve or even eliminate your child's GI issues. I strongly encourage you to take your child to a registered dietitian for professional advice and help in implementing the dietary modifications I discuss below.

Step 1: Make Appropriate Dietary Modifications

Making sure your child is getting enough fiber and water in his diet and limiting his consumption of fruit juice will promote normal daily bowel movements, which is the first basic step in healing his gut problems. Autistic children tend to accept a very limited variety of foods, so their fiber intake is usually inadequate. Refer back to page 29 in Step 2 for details on how much fiber and water (page 37) your child should have. Appendix 2 on page 216 provides a list of high-fiber foods you can offer your child. If your child has feeding problems and is unwilling or unable to eat more high-fiber foods, you may need to add a fiber supplement to his diet. However, it's important that you consult with a registered dietitian or a gastroenterologist before starting your child on a fiber product. If your child has an intestinal obstruction, fecal impaction, or narrowing of the gastrointestinal tract, a fiber supplement could cause an impaction of stool in the colon. You should also consult a registered dietitian or gastroenterologist if your child has low muscle tone. He may be unable to push stool through his lower gastrointestinal tract, and adding too much dietary fiber or a fiber supplement to his diet could result in a stool impaction.

When adding fiber to your child's diet, it's important to go slowly and make sure he's getting enough water in his diet before you increase his fiber. Your child should be drinking at most one cup of fruit juice a day, especially if he has loose stools. If he's got chronic constipation, offer him pear or apple juice, which will help to increase the water content of his stools and the frequency of his bowel movements. Prune juice is also a great choice for constipation because it contains **dihydroxyphenyl isatin**, a natural laxative substance that promotes bowel movements. I recommend mixing one to two ounces of prune juice into pear or apple juice on a daily basis.

Step 2: Try Basic Supplements

Basic supplements, such as **probiotics**, **anti-fungals**, and **digestive enzymes**, play a major role in healing your child's GI tract. The right combination of these basic supplements will support and maintain a healthy balance of naturally occurring microorganisms in your child's gastrointestinal tract.

Probiotics

The GI tract contains "good bacteria," "bad bacteria," and yeast, all of which must be maintained at an ideal balance in order to support the immune system and the production of certain vitamins and digestive enzymes. Research shows that children with autism have significant imbalances in their upper and lower gut microflora. A study published in the *Journal of Medical Microbiology* in 2005 indicated that severe gastrointestinal problems in children with autism may be due to an imbalance of the gut microflora, and that rebalancing the microflora may help to alleviate gastrointestinal disorders common in autistic children. Probiotics, which are live microorganisms that are similar to the beneficial "good bacteria" found in the gut, can help improve the microflora balance in your child's gastrointestinal tract. Probiotic supplements also work to accomplish the following:

- enhance the immune system
- decrease the frequency of acute and chronic diarrhea
- create better-formed stools
- improve dermatitis and eczema
- maintain remission in ulcerative colitis and Crohn's disease
- improve integrity of the gut barrier
- decrease GI symptoms, gut inflammation, and intestinal permeability

Most often, the bacteria used for probiotics come from two groups, *Lactobacillus* or *Bifidobacterium*. Within each group, there are different species (for example, *Lactobacillus acidophilus, Lactobacillus rhamnosus, Bifidobacterium infantis,* and *Bifidobacterium lactis*), and within each species there are different strains (or varieties). *Bifidobacterium*, especially *Bifidobacterium lactis*, is the most prevalent bacteria found in breastfed babies, making it the better supplement choice for infants and young children. *Saccha-*

romyces boulardii are yeasts that have probiotic properties and are often used in conjunction along with other probiotic supplements.

Probiotic supplements come in capsule, powder, chewable, and liquid form, making them easy for most autistic kids to ingest. If you choose a liquid probiotic supplement, be aware that it has a much shorter shelf life than the capsules, chewables, and powders. You can find probiotic supplements at most pharmacies, supermarkets, and health food stores, or they can be ordered online. (For instance, Kirkman offers a wide variety of high-quality probiotic supplements on its Web site www.kirkmangroup.com, or you can call toll-free at 800-245-8282.) When choosing one for your child, make sure it has at least 5 billion colony-forming units (CFU) per dose, as that's the minimum amount of CFU recommended by the Natural Health Products Directorate of Canada for a beneficial effect. Also be sure that your child takes the probiotic every day. Studies show that once a probiotic supplement is discontinued from the diet, the GI microflora returns to its presupplementation levels. I often recommend Culturelle, a well-known probiotic supplement that contains *Lactobacillus rhamnosus GG*, a specific strain with many well-documented health benefits. It's guaranteed to deliver a minimum of 10 billion CFU in each capsule and survive the strong acid of the stomach. (For a probiotic supplement to be effective, it must be able to survive the stomach acid so it can be delivered and colonize in the small intestines and colon.) It's also good to know that probiotic supplements often contain *fructooligosaccharides* (FOS), which is a nondigestable carbohydrate. FOS is considered a **prebiotic** because it promotes the growth of *Lactobacilli* and *Bifidobacteria*.

Antifungals

Herbs and natural food sources that have antifungal properties are often used in conjunction with probiotics. They help support a healthy balance of intestinal bacteria and yeast by keeping *Candida albican* yeast growth under control. Unlike probiotics, your child should not take an antifungal product on a daily basis. Antifungal products are typically taken for a short period of time just to assist in healing your child's GI tract, and then they're discontinued. Antifungal products contain herbs such as pau d'arco and other natural food sources that have antifungal properties such as garlic extract, grapefruit seed extract, and caprylic acid. Although most herbs are free of known side effects, there may be potential contraindications, precautions, and adverse reactions to consider, especially for children, pregnant women, and nursing mothers. You should talk to a registered dietitian or a nutrition-oriented physician for specific recommendations for your child. Some good antifungal products on the market are Yeast Fighters, manufactured by TwinLab, and YeastAid by Kirkman.

Digestive Enzymes

Digestive enzymes are secreted in the mouth, stomach, and small intestines to break down food so the body can absorb and utilize the nutrients. Studies have indicated that some autistic children have low levels of intestinal carbohydrate digestive enzymes, so a digestive enzyme supplement with meals may help them better digest their food and improve GI symptoms such as bloating, gas, diarrhea, and constipation.

The body produces different digestive enzymes to break down different types of food, so I recommend that you select a basic multispectrum digestive enzyme product that contains a blend of several different digestive enzymes. This will ensure your child will be able to handle a wide range of foods. Some examples of important digestive enzymes you should look for include the following:

- protease—breaks down protein into amino acids

- lipase—breaks down fats

- amylase—breaks down carbohydrate

- lactase—breaks down lactose into glucose and galactose

- sucrase—breaks down sucrose into glucose and fructose

There are also specialty digestive enzyme products available with higher potency levels as well as products formulated to target specific macronutrients, such as protein, fat, or carbohydrate. However, you should consult with a registered dietitian before choosing a higher potency or specially formulated product for your child. Over-the-counter digestive enzymes are usually plant-derived, well tolerated, and come in capsule form. If your child can't swallow a capsule, pull the capsule apart and mix the powder into a small amount of food or beverage at the beginning of his meal. Digestive enzyme products don't require a prescription from a physician and can be purchased at most pharmacies, supermarkets, and health food stores or ordered online. Kirkman offers a wide variety of basic, higher potency, and specially formulated digestive enzyme products (www.kirkmangroup.com).

Step 3: Consider Trying Advanced Supplements

It's worthwhile to talk with a pediatric registered dietitian and/or a gastroenterologist about trying your child on therapeutic levels of omega-3 fatty acids and glutamine to combat his gastrointestinal problems.

As you read earlier in this chapter, a significant number of children with autism have inflammation throughout their GI tract. Omega-3 fatty acids have natural anti-inflammatory properties, and research suggests that omega-3 fatty acid supplements may reduce the pain and inflammation associated with inflammatory bowel diseases such as Crohn's disease and ulcerative colitis. If your child has severe gastrointestinal symptoms or if the gastroenterologist has identified any gastrointestinal inflammation, a therapeutic level of omega-3 fatty acids for a short period of time may be a good option for him. Keep in mind that it's very important you consult a registered dietitian or physician before giving your child a therapeutic level because there are potential health risks associated with taking too much omega-3 fatty acids. (See Step 4 for more information on the benefits and risks of omega-3 fatty acids.)

Glutamine is an amino acid necessary for brain, immune, and gastrointestinal functions. One of its most important roles is to help protect the lining of the gastrointestinal tract known as the **mucosa**. Recent research studies have linked glutamine to several other GI health benefits, such as aiding in the maintenance of the gut barrier, promoting intestinal cell growth, promoting healing of the mucosa, inhibiting the growth of "bad bacteria" in the gut, improving diarrhea, and reducing the symptoms of inflammatory bowel diseases.

Glutamine is manufactured by the body, but it's also found in many dietary sources, such as beef, pork, chicken, fish, eggs, milk, dairy products, cabbage, spinach, and parsley. If your child has a very poor diet or suffers from certain medical conditions, infections, or prolonged stress, his glutamine level may be depleted and he could benefit from a glutamine supplement.

Glutamine supplements are generally labeled as L-glutamine and are sold as an individual supplement and as part of a protein supplement. They are available in capsule, tablet, powder, and liquid form. There's no RDA for glutamine, so you need to talk to your child's physician about proper dosage. The physician may order a serum amino acid lab test to determine if your child has any amino acid deficiencies before recommending a glutamine supplement. It's important to avoid a situation where your child is getting too much glutamine because excess glutamine is converted to glutamate and ammonia, which are neurotoxic in high concentrations.

Step 4: Identify and Eliminate Problematic Foods

Common gastrointestinal symptoms such as reflux, vomiting, abdominal pain, abdominal distension, gaseousness, loose stools, diarrhea, and chronic constipation are indications that your child may have an allergy, sensitivity, or intolerance to one or more foods. The most common food allergies among children are cow's milk, wheat, egg, soy, peanuts, and tree nuts. Problematic foods can have a huge impact on your child's overall health, gut function, brain function, feeding, and behavior, so it's crucial to identify and eliminate them from his diet. The good news is that if your child's GI symptoms are indeed being caused by one or more problematic foods, you'll quickly see a significant improvement in his symptoms once the foods are eliminated.

The best way to identify problematic foods for your child is through the Elimination/Challenge Diet, which I discuss in detail in Step 7. The Gluten Free Casein Free Diet (GFCF) is also an elimination/challenge diet, but it's specifically used to determine if gluten and casein are a problem for your child. In my clinical practice, I've had great success with the GFCF Diet and believe it's one of the most effective dietary treatments to improve an autistic child's GI symptoms. Turn to Step 8 on page 103 for an in-depth discussion on this diet.

MEDICAL TREATMENT

If your child still has GI symptoms after working with a registered dietitian and trying the basic nutritional interventions, his physician will need to refer him to a pediatric gastroenterologist. A pediatric gastroenterologist will examine your child for more serious GI disorders, such as gastroesophageal reflux disease (GERD), eosinophilic gastrointestinal disorders (EGID), celiac disease, **lactose intolerance**, sucrose or fructose malabsorption, fat malabsortion, bacteria overgrowth, inflammatory bowel disease (IBD), abnormal anatomy of the intestinal tract, and parasites. The gastroenterologist may have to perform certain procedures to make his diagnosis, such as an abdominal X-ray, a gastric-emptying study, an upper GI endoscopy, colonoscopy, or a pH probe. He'll also order a number of laboratory tests to rule out biomedical abnormalities that could be contributing to your child's GI symptoms, such as:

- Thyroid Panel, T3, T4, TSH (this test checks for hypothyroidism, which contributes to constipation; and hyperthyroidism, which contributes to diarrhea)

- Comprehensive Metabolic Panel (this test checks for hypercalcemia and hypokalemia, both of which contribute to constipation)

- Complete Blood Count (this test checks for iron deficiency anemia)

- Celiac Disease Panel (this test checks for celiac disease, which contributes to both constipation and diarrhea)

- Blood Lead (this test checks for abnormally high lead levels, which contribute to constipation)

- Serum Carnitine (this test checks for a carnitine deficiency, which contributes to constipation)

- Stool Analysis (this test checks for parasites, harmful bacteria, and fat malabsorption)

The results of the testing will help the gastroenterologist recommend the appropriate medical treatment, which may include medication and additional dietary interventions.

PROJECT NO. 6:

Take the following quiz to determine if your child is suffering from GI disorder symptoms:

As an infant, did your child have any of the following?

Gastroesophageal Reflux Disease (GERD)	_____ No	_____ Yes
Reflux	_____ No	_____ Yes
Projectile vomiting	_____ No	_____ Yes
Sensitivity to cow's-milk–based infant formula	_____ No	_____ Yes
Required a special infant formula	_____ No	_____ Yes

Does your child currently have any of the following?

Bloated stomach	_____ No	_____ Yes
Stomach aches	_____ No	_____ Yes
Gaseousness	_____ No	_____ Yes
Chronic constipation	_____ No	_____ Yes
Chronic diarrhea	_____ No	_____ Yes
Loose stools	_____ No	_____ Yes
Rarely has a normal formed stool	_____ No	_____ Yes
Visible undigested food in stool	_____ No	_____ Yes

Does your child have any of the following behavioral issues?

Mealtime tantrums	_____ No	_____ Yes
Consumes a limited variety of foods	_____ No	_____ Yes
Refuses to eat	_____ No	_____ Yes

If you answered "yes" to at least one of the infant and child questions, or if your child has one or more chronic GI symptoms, you should talk to a registered dietitian about basic nutritional interventions that can help.

Next, get a referral to a pediatric gastroenterologist for further testing if your child's GI symptoms persist after implementing the dietitian's recommendations.

Autism and gastrointestinal disorders often go hand in hand, and GI symptoms can be a major contributing factor to your child's behavioral issues, feeding problems, and other autistic symptoms. Identifying and treating undiagnosed GI disorders is a critical part of treating your child's autism. Once you've completed Step 6, you should see a significant improvement in your child's autistic symptoms. If your child suffers from a food allergy, sensitivity, or intolerance, Step 7 will show you exactly how to identify and eliminate any foods that are creating a problem.

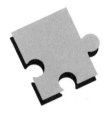

STEP 7

Identify and Treat Food Allergies

Food allergies are becoming a serious concern for American children. An estimated 6 to 8 percent of children under the age of three suffer from food allergies, and the numbers continue to rise. There's also a growing body of evidence that shows there's an increased incidence of food allergies among children with autism and related disorders such as ADHD compared to the general population of children. Autistic children may be more vulnerable to food allergies because of abnormalities in their digestive and/or immune systems. Research also supports a link between food allergies and behavioral problems, though the medical community has been hesitant to acknowledge this. Understanding how food allergies may be affecting your child and eliminating problematic foods from his diet is a critical component of his comprehensive treatment plan.

THE FOOD ALLERGY–BEHAVIOR CONNECTION

Food allergies don't cause children to have autism or other related disorders, but they do affect children with these conditions more than typically developing children. This is because children with autism, Asperger's, PDD, ADHD, and ADD share a common problem—they tend to have some degree of sensory integration dysfunction. You may remember from Step 5 that children with sensory integration dysfunction have trouble responding appropriately to sensory information from their environment. They're more sensitive, become easily overwhelmed, and may overreact (or underreact) to auditory, visual, and tactile stimulation. If your child already has sensory issues, allergy symptoms like itchy skin, hives, eczema, runny nose, sneezing, and itchy, tearing eyes will stress his sensory system further, making it even more difficult for him to function normally. The combination of food allergies and sensory issues can hinder your child's ability to sit still, concentrate, maintain focus, process information, learn, control his impulses and behavior, and interact with his teachers and therapists. Relieving your child of food allergy symptoms will lessen the sensory burden he has to deal with, which will improve his behavior.

Autistic children are unique because they're often unable to verbally express the physical discomfort and pain they feel from food allergy symptoms. If your child is nonverbal or has an expressive language delay, he can't tell you if he feels nausea, abdominal pain, chest pain from reflux, or headaches. Instead, your child has to "communicate" physical pain through his behavior, such as head banging, tantrums, irritability, and food refusal. This is crucial for you to know because these behaviors are very often mistaken for typical autistic behavioral problems instead of behaviors caused by undiagnosed food allergies.

WHAT IS A FOOD ALLERGY?

Although many people use the terms "allergy," "sensitivity," and "intolerance" interchangeably, they really describe three different food-related conditions.

An allergy is defined as an adverse immune response to a food protein. A food allergy occurs when the immune system mistakenly identifies a specific protein found in food as a harmful substance and defends against it. Food allergies are classified according to how the immune system responds and are split into two categories: **IgE mediated** and **non-IgE mediated**.

IgE Mediated Food Allergy

With an IgE mediated food allergy, the immune system triggers immunoglobulin E (IgE) antibodies to bind with the food protein (also known as the **allergen**) activating cells throughout the body to release **histamine** and other chemicals. These chemicals cause inflammation and a range of allergic reactions throughout the body, affecting your child's respiratory system, gastrointestinal tract, skin, eyes, ears, nose, and/or throat.

IgE mediated reactions can be either immediate or delayed. Immediate reactions generally occur within seconds up to two hours after eating the offending food. Delayed reactions occur between two and forty-eight hours after eating the offending food. IgE mediated food allergies can be detected through special testing (see page 96 for more information).

Some people experience a more severe allergic reaction called **anaphylaxis**, where they have difficulty breathing, a rapid pulse, dizziness, and enter a state of shock with a rapid drop in blood pressure. Anaphylaxis is potentially life-threatening and requires immediate medical attention.

Non-IgE Mediated Food Allergy

A non-IgE mediated food allergy triggers a different kind of immune system response. The immune system responds directly to a food protein, causing the release of certain chemicals. This leads to inflammation that causes a variety of milder reactions throughout the body, primarily in the gastrointestinal tract. GI symptoms include chronic diarrhea, loose stools, constipation, nausea, vomiting, reflux, bloating, and abdominal pain. Non-IgE mediated food allergies can cause the development of serious gastrointestinal conditions, such as **food protein–induced enterocolitis** (the inflammation of the small and large intestines), **gastroenteritis** (the inflammation of the stomach and small intestines), and **esophagitis** (the inflammation of the esophagus).

Many people don't realize that IgE mediated food allergies are responsible for only about 5 percent of adverse food reactions; the other 95 percent are caused by non-IgE mediated food allergies, sensitivities, and intolerances. Unfortunately, standard food allergy testing can identify only IgE mediated allergies. This is why an elimination/challenge diet is so important. It's the only way to detect the other 95 percent of adverse food reactions that affect so many children. Sadly, most practitioners in the traditional medical community focus only on that 5 percent of testable reactions and overlook the significance of non-IgE mediated food allergies. This leaves countless children undiagnosed, untreated, and continuing to suffer with gastrointestinal and other physical problems that negatively affect their behavior and ability to function normally. Studies have demonstrated that when non-IgE mediated food allergies are treated in autistic children, their behavioral issues improve. Research conducted by Dr. Harumi Jyonouchi and published in *Neuropsychobiology* in 2002 and 2005 and the *Journal of Pediatrics* in 2005 indicated that autistic children who had a non-IgE mediated immune response to gluten, casein, and soy experienced behavioral improvements when placed on a gluten, casein, and soy elimination diet. Clearly, children with non-IgE mediated food allergies will never have the opportunity to reach their full potential until their allergies are identified and treated.

The symptoms of a non-IgE mediated food allergy generally develop several hours to days after eating the offending food. This type of allergy is much harder to identify because currently there are no reliable diagnostic tests available to detect it. Since a non-IgE mediated food allergy reaction does not involve an IgE antibody, the standard RAST and prick skin tests are not useful. The only way you can determine if your child has a non-IgE mediated allergy to specific foods is to put him on an elimination/challenge diet. (See page 98 for information on implementing this diet.)

Mixed IgE and Non-IgE Mediated Food Allergy

Some kids suffer from a mix of IgE and non-IgE mediated food allergies, especially those who have eosinophilic esophagitis (EE), eosinophilic gastroenteritis (EG), and eosinophilic colitis (EC). In this case, a blood test and skin prick test will identify only some of your child's allergies, and an elimination/challenge diet must be used to identify the rest.

The Most Common Food Allergies

The following foods are responsible for 90 percent of allergic reactions:

- milk
- wheat
- soy
- eggs
- peanuts
- tree nuts (pecans, walnuts, almonds, cashews, hazel, and Brazil nuts)
- fish
- shellfish

Milk, wheat, soy, eggs, and peanuts are the most common food allergens in children under the age of three. Allergic reactions to fish and shellfish are more common in adults, and allergic reactions to fruits and vegetables also tend to occur later in life.

WHAT IS A FOOD SENSITIVITY?

A food sensitivity is a general term used to describe an abnormal reaction to a food or food additive. A food sensitivity is different from a food allergy because the reaction doesn't involve the immune system. Food sensitivity symptoms are virtually identical to those of an allergy, but they tend to be much milder. If your child is sensitive to a particular food, he's most likely reacting to the artificial food additives in the food as opposed to the food itself. The following artificial additives are the most common culprits:

- sulfites
- aspartame

- MSG
- yellow dye No. 5
- preservatives (BHT and BHA)

As you may recall from Step 1, you should eliminate all unnecessary artificial food additives from your child's diet, such as artificial colors, artificial flavors, preservatives, and artificial sweeteners.

WHAT IS A FOOD INTOLERANCE?

Similar to a food sensitivity, a food intolerance doesn't involve the immune system. It occurs when something in a food irritates a person's digestive system or when a person has too few or none of the enzymes that enable him to properly digest, or break down, a food. For instance, if your child has too few or is missing the enzymes necessary to break down carbohydrates in the small intestines, the carbohydrates pass undigested into the colon where they ferment and produce excess gas, bloating, abdominal cramps, and diarrhea.

The three carbohydrates that make up the most common food intolerances are lactose, sucrose, and fructose. You're probably familiar with the term lactose intolerance, which is the most common carbohydrate intolerance. If your child is lactose intolerant, his body doesn't have sufficient levels of lactase, the enzyme that metabolizes lactose, the carbohydrate in milk. A lactase deficiency will render your child unable to digest the lactose in milk, so lactose passes from the small intestines undigested into the colon and causes abdominal symptoms. Lactose intolerance can be identified with an **oral tolerance test** or a **hydrogen breath test**.

WHY DOES YOUR CHILD HAVE A FOOD ALLERGY?

I mentioned earlier that experts believe autistic children may be more vulnerable to food allergies because of abnormalities in their digestive and/or immune systems. In a normally functioning digestive system, digestive enzymes break down the protein in foods into small, single molecules called amino acids. The amino acids then pass through the lining of the gastrointestinal wall (also known as the gut-blood barrier) into the bloodstream and are used throughout the body as needed. The junction between cells in the gastrointestinal wall are tightly bound and act as a barrier to ensure only small, single molecules such as amino acids, vitamins, and minerals are allowed into the bloodstream. It's *theorized* that autistic children with gastrointestinal and/or immune system abnormalities have abnormally increased permeability (also known as "leaky gut syndrome") of their gut-blood barrier that allows large, intact protein molecules to pass into the bloodstream. This triggers their immune system to overreact to an otherwise harmless food, identifying the protein molecule as a foreign particle and initiating a defense. As the protein molecule circulates throughout the body, cells react by releasing histamine, **cytokines**, **interleukins**, and other chemicals that trigger inflammation and allergy symptoms.

If your child suffers from one or more of the following symptoms, a food allergy may be to blame:

Ears—otitis media (ear infections)

Nose—nasal congestion, sneezing, runny nose

Eyes—tearing, puffy eyes, dark circles under eyes

Oral—swelling of lips, tongue, mouth, and throat

Skin—hives, eczema, red cheeks, itching

Respiratory—difficulty breathing, cough, wheezing, asthma

Intestinal—reflux, vomiting, nausea, abdominal pain, diarrhea, constipation

Neurological—headache, migraine, and behavioral problems such as tantrums, irritability, and hyperactivity

HOW TO IDENTIFY PROBLEMATIC FOODS FOR YOUR CHILD

If you suspect your child suffers from a food allergy, sensitivity, or intolerance, take him to see a board-certified allergist for a definitive diagnosis. The allergist will perform a physical exam, take down your child's medical and dietary history, and order diagnostic tests to rule out other medical conditions. Then he'll order a RAST and skin prick test to help identify an IgE mediated allergy and will probably conduct a physician-supervised oral food challenge to confirm positive test results. He'll also likely suggest a short-term elimination/challenge diet to identify any non-IgE mediated allergies.

RAST Test

If your child is older than one year, the allergist will perform a radioallergosorbent test (RAST) to help identify food allergies. The RAST is a blood test that detects IgE antibodies to a particular food. The allergist might also perform a CAP RAST or CAP

System FEIA, which is a specific type of RAST test that indicates the level of IgE anti-bodies present for each allergen. This can help predict how severe your child's reaction to a problematic food will be.

It's important to know that the RAST does have some limitations. About half of the time, the RAST returns a false-positive test result. This means that the RAST may detect an IgE antibody in your child and indicate a positive result for a particular food, but your child isn't actually allergic to the food. This can lead to unnecessary elimination of foods from your child's diet. Usually, if the RAST results indicate a positive reaction to a food, the allergist will conduct an oral food challenge under his supervision. Your child will be given capsules filled with the suspected allergen and watched for symptoms of an allergic reaction to determine if he's really allergic to that food. Once the allergist has reached a definite diagnosis, the food will be eliminated from your child's diet.

The RAST also returns a high percentage of false-negative results, which means that the test may not detect IgE mediated food allergies your child *does* have. Ultimately, the RAST is nothing more than a helpful screening test. It's not intended to provide a definitive diagnosis of food allergies. Also, the RAST can't detect non-IgE mediated food allergies.

Skin Prick Test

The skin prick test is also used to help identify IgE mediated food allergies in children older than one year. First, a small amount of a suspected **food allergen** is placed on your child's skin or on a testing device. Then the testing device pricks through the top layer of your child's skin and inserts the allergen under the skin. If your child is allergic, a hive will form at that spot.

Like the RAST, the skin prick test also has some limitations. Its false-positive rate is more than 50 percent, which is especially problematic for children with skin issues, such as eczema. The good news is that the skin prick test has a very low incidence of false-negative results; if your child tests negative for an allergen, there's a 95 percent chance he's *not* allergic to that food. Like the RAST, the skin prick test is nothing more than a helpful screening test and is not intended to provide a definitive diagnosis of food allergies. The skin prick test also can't detect non-IgE mediated food allergies.

Don't Forget about Airborne Allergies

Some of the symptoms your child is experiencing may be caused by airborne allergies, such as pet dander, dust mites, mold, tree, weed, and grass pollens.

When the allergist orders blood drawn to complete a RAST for food allergens, ask that he also test for common airborne allergens so they too can be identified and treated.

Elimination/Challenge Diet

The elimination/challenge diet is used to rule out false-positive and false-negative results from the RAST and skin prick tests. It's also the only method to identify non-IgE mediated food allergies. If you want to put your child on an elimination/challenge diet, be sure to discuss with an allergist which foods can safely be challenged at home without medical supervision. A short-term elimination/challenge diet involves two basic steps:

1. ***Eliminate the suspected food from your child's diet for two weeks.***
   This will give your child's allergy symptoms time to subside. If your child has EE, EG, and/or EC, suspected food allergens may need to be eliminated for eight to twelve weeks to achieve symptom improvement. The first foods you should eliminate are those that had positive RAST and/or skin prick test results. If both of these tests came back negative, start with the foods that tend to be the most likely culprits: milk, wheat, soy, eggs, peanuts, nuts, fish, and shellfish.

2. ***Challenge your child with an eliminated food.***
   Once your child has been off a suspected allergenic food for the appropriate period of time, reintroduce the food to his diet for one week. Watch to see if his allergy symptoms recur. If you eliminated more than one food, add back one food at a time each week.

It's very important that you consult with a registered dietitian about putting your child on this diet. These steps are very general, and a dietitian can adapt them to meet your child's unique needs. Special issues such as consuming a very limited variety of foods or refusing to accept new foods will impact the number of foods that can be eliminated from your child's diet at a given time. An elimination/challenge diet is more complicated for autistic children who have a feeding problem or self-limit their diet to foods consisting exclusively of milk and wheat products. In this situation, the best approach is usually to address your child's feeding problem first before eliminating any foods from his diet.

There are many other diagnostic allergy tests available, but most are questionable and considered very controversial. Of these tests, the one most commonly used for autistic children is the IgG ELISA blood test, which tests for more than one hundred different foods. The American Academy of Allergy and Immunology's position is that this test is lacking and not an acceptable method of diagnosing food allergies. Most mainstream physicians and allergists also claim there is no value to this test. However, physicians who practice complementary medicine claim that the IgG ELISA test identifies delayed food allergies and is useful in treating autism, hyperactivity, arthritis, fatigue, headaches, and other conditions. Several research studies have been published in the *Scandinavian Journal of Gastroenterology* and the *Journal of the American College of Nutrition* since 2004 that indicate that food elimination based on positive IgG ELISA test results strongly correlates with significant improvement in individuals diagnosed with Irritable Bowel Syndrome (IBS). It appears that the IgG ELISA blood test may at least be helpful in treating gastrointestinal symptoms, which is a major problem for autistic children.

NUTRITIONAL TREATMENT FOR FOOD ALLERGIES

If your child has been diagnosed with a food allergy, getting professional help from a registered dietitian is critical. The dietitian will guide you through the nutrition therapy component of treating food allergies, which involves nutritional interventions to heal the gastrointestinal tract, elimination of allergenic foods, identifying and resolving any nutrient deficiencies, and assessing your child's growth.

Unfortunately, I've found that when a child is diagnosed with one or more food allergies, his parents are not referred to a registered dietitian. Instead, the allergist sends them home with a long list of foods to avoid. The parents do their best to eliminate the allergenic foods, but often they don't know what foods to substitute, causing their child's diet to become extremely limited and nutritionally inadequate. This is especially a problem for autistic children who often already have a very limited diet. Eliminating common foods such as milk, wheat, eggs, and soy can have a major impact on the nutritional quality of your child's diet. Studies indicate that children with two or more food allergies have low intakes of calcium, iron, vitamin D, vitamin E, and zinc and are at higher risk for decreased growth in height. Make sure you get a dietitian referral from your child's physician and/or allergist, and don't attempt to implement this diet on your own.

Healing the GI Tract

Healing your child's GI tract is an important component of treating food allergies, especially for autistic children with gastrointestinal disorders. As I mentioned earlier, your child's gut-blood barrier may have abnormal increased permeability (also referred to as "leaky"), allowing large, intact protein molecules into the bloodstream and triggering the immune system to overreact. In this case, healing his GI tract before starting an elimination diet is a more effective food allergy treatment than the elimination diet alone. Once your child's GI tract is healed, his intestinal permeability will become normal, his gastrointestinal inflammation will decrease, and his digestive system will be restored to good health. Turn back to Step 6 on page 83 for details on the three important nutritional interventions that will heal your child's gut: dietary treatment (adequate fiber and water); basic supplements (probiotics, antifungals, and digestive enzymes); and advanced supplements (therapeutic levels of omega-3 fatty acids and glutamine).

The Elimination Diet

An elimination diet seems like it should be pretty straightforward—your child will cut allergenic foods from his diet. However, this diet can be very complicated, especially if your child has multiple food allergies. A registered dietitian will help you:

- understand how to avoid allergenic foods,
- find appropriate substitutions for eliminated foods,
- handle eating situations away from home,
- make meal modifications for school lunch,
- read food labels,
- avoid cross-contamination of allergenic foods and safe foods,
- locate local and mail-order sources for allergen-free products,
- replace the nutrients lost from the eliminated foods.

Studies indicate that approximately 44 percent of children younger than three years of age with allergies to milk, wheat, soy, and eggs outgrow their food allergy within one to seven years. (Allergies to peanuts, tree nuts, fish, and shellfish are often lifelong, and food allergies that develop after the age of three years are less likely to be outgrown.) If you remove known allergenic foods from your child's diet, it actually improves his chances of outgrowing his allergies. In light of this, it's a good idea for you to re-challenge your child after one year on the elimination diet to see if he's still reactive to the allergenic foods. If his allergy symptoms don't return, you can add the foods back into his diet. If your child does react to the food re-challenge, continue to avoid the allergenic foods and do a re-challenge on an annual basis. If your child's allergic reaction symptoms to problematic foods are severe, consult with an allergist before doing a food re-challenge.

An excellent resource of educational materials and more detailed information related to food allergies, including list of foods and ingredients to avoid, can be found on the Food Allergy and Anaphylaxis Network (FAAN) Web site at www.foodallergy.org.

Ben's Story

Four-year-old Ben was diagnosed with pervasive developmental disorder—not otherwise specified (PDD-NOS), sensory integration dysfunction, and delayed speech. At the age of two, Ben's mother suspected he had problems with certain foods. She reported that after eating wheat products he became agitated and more hyperactive. She also reported that Ben had stomach aches and didn't participate in his therapy sessions after eating lunch. Instead he would lie flat and outstretched, pressing his stomach into the floor, and would refuse to get up. He also had chronic diarrhea, eczema, wheezing, and a constant runny nose. When Ben tried peanuts for the first time, his lips swelled up, so Ben's mom took him to an allergist. The RAST came back positive for multiple food allergies—peanut, soybean, wheat, corn, and egg white. He also tested positive for dust mites, cat and dog dander, grass, and ragweed. Ben's mom told me she had been advised to eliminate peanuts, soy, wheat, corn, and eggs from Ben's diet; provided with and instructed on how to use an **EPIPEN**; given prescriptions for Rhinocort nasal spray, topical cortisol steroid cream, and an oral antihistamine medication; and she was given several handouts with lists of foods to avoid. A physician-supervised oral food challenge or short-term elimination/challenge diet was not conducted to confirm the food allergies. Ben's mom was not referred to a registered dietitian to help her implement Ben's long-term elimination diet. She told me it was extremely difficult trying to eliminate so many foods from Ben's diet and that she was feeling overwhelmed and frustrated. She chose to focus on the elimination of peanuts and allowed Ben to continue to eat the other foods. Ben continued to suffer with behavioral problems after meals, stomach aches, and diarrhea. He got partial relief from the eczema, wheezing, and runny nose from medications his doctor prescribed.

Ben was four when I began to work with him. I referred him to another board-certified allergist, who assessed him comprehensively and took a more holistic approach to treating both his airborne and food allergies. The allergist supervised an oral food challenge, which indicated that Ben had an immediate reaction to peanuts. A short-term elimination/challenge diet for wheat, soy, corn, and eggs indicted that Ben reacted to wheat and soy, but corn and eggs were not a problem. Ben's long-term elimination diet consisted of avoiding peanuts, wheat, and soy. Ben's symptoms of diarrhea, eczema, wheezing, stomach aches, and behavioral problems after meals all disappeared. He was able to stop using the Rhinocort nasal spray and topical cortisol steroid cream and instead began using an oral antihistamine occasionally for seasonal airborne allergies. After one year on the elimination diet, Ben was re-challenged with wheat and soy. This time he was able to tolerate soy, but wheat continued to trigger allergic reactions. It was recommended that Ben continue a wheat and peanut elimination diet. His mom reports that Ben is now free of both allergy symptoms and medications and is a healthier and happier child.

PROJECT NO. 7: IDENTIFY AND TREAT YOUR CHILD'S FOOD ALLERGIES

1. Look at the list of food allergy symptoms on page 96. Does your child experience any of these symptoms on a frequent or chronic basis? If so, schedule an appointment with a board-certified allergist to identify IgE mediated food allergies using RAST and skin prick tests. Confirm positive results with a physician-supervised oral food challenge or short-term elimination/challenge diet as recommended by the allergist. Then you should find a registered dietitian who can help you implement a short-term elimination/challenge diet to identify possible non-IgE mediated food allergies.

2. Once your child is diagnosed with a particular food allergy, work with a dietitian to avoid that food using a long-term elimination diet.

As you can see, diagnosing food allergies is complicated, test results are difficult to interpret, current blood lab and skin tests aren't always accurate, some allergy tests are controversial, and treatment is challenging. Even so, identifying and treating your child's food allergies has enormous benefits. He will experience a wide range of physical, gastrointestinal, and neurological (including behavioral) improvements. Avoiding problematic foods is a critical step in nutritional treatment of your child's autism. The next step is to consider some of the special elimination diets that are commonly recommended for autistic children.

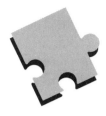

STEP 8

Consider Putting Your Child
on a Special Elimination Diet

Elimination diets, especially the Gluten Free Casein Free (GFCF) diet, are very popular in the autism community. Parents have long claimed that these diets are effective in relieving autistic symptoms. However, there's very little evidence-based scientific research out there that supports or refutes these claims. These dietary interventions are considered controversial and usually not supported by the medical community. That said, this doesn't necessarily mean that one of these elimination diets won't be helpful for your child. In this chapter, I focus mainly on the GFCF diet, as my experience has shown this to be the most effective diet for autistic kids. You'll learn about the theory behind the GFCF diet, the potential benefits, and how to transition your child onto it. I also discuss the Specific Carbohydrate Diet (SCD), the rotation diet, the antifungal diet, and the Feingold Diet. It's very important that you don't try to implement any elimination diet on your own. Find a knowledgeable registered dietitian who can work with you to ensure the diet is implemented properly, show you how to assess the diet's effectiveness, and help you replace lost nutrients from eliminated foods so you're not compromising your child's nutritional health.

THE GLUTEN FREE CASEIN FREE DIET (GFCF DIET)

The GFCF diet is the single most common elimination diet recommended for autistic children. It's not considered a "cure" for autism, but rather a means to relieve autistic, behavioral, and gastrointestinal symptoms in autistic children. There are several theories as to why eliminating the proteins gluten (found in wheat, rye, and barley) and casein (found in milk) from the diet may be beneficial.

The Opiate Excess Theory

The link between gluten, casein, and autism was first reported by K. Reichelt, M.D., in the 1980s. Reichelt performed a study in which he analyzed the urine of autistic children and found abnormally high levels of the peptides **gliadomorphine** and **casomorphine**. Peptides, which are short chains of amino acids, are created when the digestion of proteins by enzymes is not completed. The peptide gliadomorphine results from the incomplete digestion of gluten, and casomorphine is the result of the incomplete digestion of casein. Gliadomorphine and casomorphine are referred to as **opiate peptides** because their chemical structure is similar to opiates. It's been proposed that these opiate peptides may also act similarly to opiates, depressing the central nervous system, which could precipitate or aggravate autistic symptoms. Thus the "opiate excess theory" was born.

Opiates naturally occur in the central nervous system (CNS), but the levels of opiate peptides that Reichelt found in the urine of autistic children were too high to have originated in the CNS. So the conclusion was that the excessive levels of gliadomorphine and casomorphine peptides came from an outside source—the incomplete digestion of gluten and casein found in foods. Since peptides are generally too large to pass through the gastrointestinal wall into the bloodstream, the theory suggests that they got into the blood through a "leaky gut." In other words, the linings of the autistic children's intestinal tracts were too permeable, allowing the opiate peptides to slip through the gut-blood barrier into the bloodstream. The peptides were then transported to the kidneys and excreted out of the body in urine. The theory goes on to say that if some of the opiate peptides were not excreted and instead stayed in the bloodstream, they could possibly cross the **blood-brain barrier (BBB)** and attach to opiate receptors in the brain. If this happened, the peptides would mimic other opiates, such as morphine, and interfere with normal brain function, resulting in autistic symptoms.

If the opiate excess theory is accurate, then removing the dietary sources of opiate peptides (gluten and casein) from your child's diet would help improve his behavioral and autistic symptoms.

The Non-IgE Mediated Food Allergy Theory

This more recent theory suggests that autistic children may be predisposed to allergic reactions to dietary proteins (gluten, casein, and soy), which leads to gastrointestinal inflammation and behavioral symptoms. Research conducted by Dr. Harami Jyonouchi indicates that while only a small percentage of autistic children tested positive for IgE-mediated food allergies via IgE RAST and skin prick tests for gluten, casein, and soy, a significant percentage of these same children experienced symptom improvement on a gluten, casein, and soy elimination diet. Jyonouchi found that autistic children had an increased proinflammatory cytokine response to gluten, casein, and soy, which indicates that these children did indeed have a non-IgE-mediated immune reaction to dietary proteins. The studies concluded that non-IgE-mediated immune reactions to gluten, casein, and soy play a role in gastrointestinal symptoms in autistic children.

SHOULD YOU PUT YOUR CHILD ON THE GFCF DIET?

As I mentioned earlier, there's very little research-based evidence that supports or refutes the effectiveness of the GFCF diet for autistic children. However, since the early 1980s, many parents have tried the diet with their autistic children, and the vast majority report positive results. According to these anecdotal reports, the GFCF diet accomplishes the following:

- relieves gastrointestinal symptoms
- helps children pass normal, formed stools
- decreases hyperactivity
- increases focus
- reduces behavioral problems
- improves speech and communication skills
- and improves sleep

Parents often ask me if there's a lab test that can tell them for sure whether their child will benefit from the GFCF diet before they start it. Unfortunately, the answer is no. Some private labs do promote a urinary peptides test that measures the level of gliadomorphine and casomorphine in urine; however, this test is very controversial and usually not recommended by medical professionals. The only sure way to know whether your child will respond positively to the GFCF diet is to try him on it, and that choice is yours alone. If you do decide to move forward, you'll need to keep your child on the diet for at least three full months for trustworthy results.

UNDERSTANDING THE BASICS

Gluten, casein, and soy (I include soy here because it's another highly allergenic dietary protein that I usually suggest eliminating as part of the GFCF diet) are found in more foods and beverages than you may think. It's really important that you're able to recognize products that may contain these proteins. The following is a rundown of the basics.

Gluten

Gluten is the protein found in wheat, barley, and rye. It gives flour its elasticity, which allows for **leavening**, and provides texture to baked products. Gluten is commonly found in breads, pasta, cereals, and baked goods. It's not found in oats, but oat is eliminated from the GFCF diet because of the high possibility of **cross contamination** by wheat, barley, or rye during its processing and distribution. Also, research indicates that **avenin**, the protein found in oats, has a peptide sequence that closely resembles wheat gluten, so cutting out oat makes sense.

Gluten is used as a stabilizing agent in food products, so it can be found in unexpected places. You'll need to read food ingredient labels carefully to identify products that may have "hidden gluten" and need to be avoided. There are some food additives that may or may not contain gluten, and you'll need to contact the manufacturer for clarification. Nonfood sources also need to be considered because gluten is often used in medications, vitamin and mineral supplements, cosmetics, and other products. Here's a list of common food products to avoid:

barley	oatmeal	triticale
bran	pasta	udon
couscous	rye	wheat
Cream of Wheat	seitan	wheat germ
farina	semolina	wheat flour
Kamut	spelt	wheat starch
malt	sprouted wheat	soy and teriyaki sauces
matzo/matzoh meal	sprouted barley	(unless labeled wheat
oats	tabbouleh	free)

These food additives *may* contain gluten, so you'll need to contact the manufacturer to find out:

emulsifiers	hydrolyzed vegetable protein (HVP)	seasonings
fillers	texturized vegetable protein (TVP)	stabilizers
flavoring	modified food starch	vegetable protein

Note: Be aware that convenience foods often use gluten-containing flours as a thickener in gravies, soups, and custards.

Here are some common nonfood sources of gluten to be aware of:

over-the-counter and prescription medications

vitamin and mineral supplements (especially tablet form)

cosmetics (lipstick, lip gloss, and lip balms)

Play-Doh

glue

And lastly, here is a list of gluten-free foods that are *safe* to include in your child's diet:

amaranth	guar gum
arrowroot	herbs
annatto	hydrogenated vegetable oil
baking soda	kasha
beans	legumes (beans, fava bean, soybean, garbanzo bean, lentils, peas, peanuts)
buckwheat	
canola oil	locust bean gum
carob	maltodextrin (from corn or rice)
cellulose gum	meat
chickpeas	fish
corn	shellfish
corn meal	game
corn starch	millet
Cream of Rice	nuts (almond, chestnut, acorn, hazelnut, walnuts, Brazil, cashew)
distilled vinegar	
eggs	popcorn
flax	potatoes
flours (nut, rice, potato, soy)	quinoa
fruit	rice
gelatin	rice products (rice cakes, pasta, bread, crackers, pasta)
grits	

(Continues)

sago

seeds (sunflower, mustard, sesame, safflower, coconut, poppy, alfalfa)

sorghum

sesame

soy

sweet potatoes

tapioca

teff

vegetables

water

xanthan gum

yams

Casein

Casein is the protein found in milk and milk products. When eliminating milk from your child's diet, you're also eliminating a major source of calcium, vitamin D, and protein, so be sure to enlist the help of a registered dietitian to assess your child's diet and recommend replacements for these key nutrients. Here's a list of common foods your child should avoid:

milk (nonfat, lowfat, skim, whole, buttermilk, dry, powdered, condensed, evaporated, malted)

butter (butterfat, butter oil, butter solids, artificial butter flavor)

caseinates (all forms)

cheese (all forms)

cheese flavor

cream

cottage cheese

curds

custard

ghee

goat's milk

half & half

ice cream

ice milk

lactoglobulin

lactalbumin

lactalbumin phosphate

lactoferrin

milk chocolate

nougat

pudding

rennet

sherbet

sour cream

whey

yogurt

Note: Whey is a different milk protein from casein, so it could be included in a casein-free diet. However, experts suggest that you avoid whey unless it clearly states on the product label that it's casein-free.

Here's a list of food products and additives that may have casein, so you should call the manufacturer for clarification:

brown sugar flavoring	natural flavoring
canned tuna	nondairy creamer
caramel flavoring	salad dressings
chocolate	sauces
commercially prepared mixes	Simplesse
high protein flour	soups
lactic acid starter culture	vegetarian nondairy cheese substitutes
margarine	whipped topping
packaged dinners	
processed meats (hot dogs, luncheon, sausage)	

Lastly, here's a list of casein-free milk substitutions you can *safely* include in your child's diet:

coconut	nuts	potato	rice	Vance's DariFree

Note: It's a good idea to buy "fortified" milk substitutions, which contain extra calcium, vitamin D, and other nutrients.

Soy

Soybean, also known as soya bean, is a type of legume. It's considered a good source of protein because it contains all nine of the essential amino acids needed to build and maintain human body tissues. Until recently, soy was used as a substitution for dairy products in the GFCF diet, Now, because of the research done by Dr. Jyonouchi (see page 93 for more on this) and the fact that soy is a common food allergen, most health-care practitioners agree that it's best to also eliminate soy while on the GFCF diet. Here's a list of common foods your child should avoid:

edamane	shoyu sauce	soy flour	soy milk
natto	soy nuts	soy sauce	soy sprouts
miso	Tamari sauce	tempeh	tofu

The following food additives may contain soy, so you'll need to contact the manufacturer to find out:

hydrolyzed vegetable protein (HVP)
lecithin
monodiglyceride
monosodium glutamate (MSG)
natural flavorings
textured vegetable protein (TVP)

GETTING YOUR CHILD STARTED

Starting an autistic child on an elimination diet must be handled very carefully. Many autistic kids' diets consists mostly of wheat, milk, and processed food products. Many have feeding problems such as refusing new foods, mealtime tantrums, and refusing to eat. So it's not as simple as just cutting out foods containing gluten and casein and replacing them with new, safe foods. Given these complications, you'll probably need to take some additional steps to prepare your child for the transition to the GFCF diet before you actually start it. I find it helpful to break it into two stages: preparing to start the diet and then the actual elimination of gluten, casein, and soy. Each stage has a progression of steps that allow you to move forward at your own comfort level.

Stage 1: Preparing to Start the GFCF Diet

Step 1: Find Professional Help. An elimination/challenge diet is considered nutrition therapy. You should recruit help from a medical professional, preferably a registered dietitian.

Step 2: Focus on the Foods Your Child Can Eat. With help from the RD, make a list of all the foods your child is allowed to eat, whether he's willing to eat them or not. You'll be surprised by how extensive your list is. Then mark which foods your child will currently eat and compile his personal "safe foods" list.

Step 3: Prepare Meals with Whole Foods That Are Naturally Gluten- and Casein-Free. Get back to the basics by preparing simpler meals using healthy, whole foods and rely less on prepackaged processed foods that contain "unsafe" ingredients. Select foods such as meat, poultry, fish, shellfish, game, eggs, dried beans and peas, nuts and seeds, fruits, vegetables, potatoes, rice, and corn.

Step 4: Buy Gluten- and Casein-Free Food Products. These days, most grocery stores have a section dedicated to special foods, including gluten- and casein-free foods. Certainly your local health food store and Whole Foods Market carry many gluten- and casein-free choices. You can also search the Internet for mail order companies that specialize in allergen-free foods and packaged pre-mixes.

Step 5: Join a Parent Support Group. It's easy to feel overwhelmed during this process, and a support group can help you work through your feelings and offer much-needed support. Also, networking with other parents of autistic children using the GFCF diet is a great way to get information, advice, and learn about other helpful resources.

Stage 2: Eliminating Gluten and Casein
Step 1: Expose Your Child to Gluten- and Casein-Free Foods in a Gradual and Non-threatening Manner. At each meal, along with the typical foods your child is willing to eat, offer him at least one gluten- and casein-free food to start the exposure process. Your child needs to see, smell, and touch a new food, even if he won't eat it yet.

If your child has serious feeding problems, such as throwing tantrums at the sight of a new food or refusing to tolerate new foods on the dinner table or his plate, you may not be able to accomplish Step 1. Serious feeding problems like these require feeding therapy from a team of professionals, as I discussed in Step 5. If this is the case for your child, gluten- and casein-free foods should be introduced during his feeding therapy sessions. You'll need to delay starting the elimination stage until his feeding problem improves, he tolerates new foods on his plate, and his diet has expanded to include eating gluten- and casein-free foods.

Step 2: Eliminate Obvious Sources of Gluten and Casein from Your Child's Diet. Identify the foods your child currently eats that are the most obvious sources of gluten and casein and replace them with a gluten- and casein-free alternative. These new, "safe" foods must also replace the vitamins, minerals, protein, and other nutrients that are lost from the eliminated foods. For example, replace cow's milk with "fortified" rice milk.

Step 3: Identify and Eliminate "Hidden" Sources of Gluten and Casein. Processed foods and prepackaged foods often contain hidden sources of gluten and casein. Read food ingredient labels closely and look for uncertain food additives that may contain gluten or casein. If you're not sure about a food product, contact the manufacturer and ask exactly what ingredients it contains. Also, look for gluten and casein in the common nonfood sources, such as medicine and vitamin and mineral supplements. Replace any unsafe products with a safe alternative.

Step 4: Fill Family, Friends, Teachers, and Caregivers in on Your Plan. You'll need to educate your child's caregivers, extended family, daycare, and school staff about the GFCF diet and request their full cooperation to implement the diet properly. It's important for you to feel confident that your child's GFCF diet is being adhered to everywhere he goes. Your child's dietitian can act as a consultant to his daycare and school cafeteria staff to ensure the menu accommodates his dietary restrictions.

Step 5: Assess Whether Your Child is a "Positive Responder" or "Nonresponder" to the Diet. A large percentage of autistic children are considered "positive responders," which means they experience symptom improvement on the GFCF diet and when gluten and/or casein is added back to their diet, the symptoms return. However, the GFCF diet doesn't help every autistic child. A "nonresponder" to the diet won't show any symptom improvement at all.

It may take some time to completely transition your child to the GFCF diet, depending on his feeding and sensory issues. Once you feel confident that you've completely eliminated gluten and casein from your child's diet, it's time to officially begin the three-month elimination phase to determine whether he's a positive responder or nonresponder. You'll need to be observant and objective and record your child's autistic, behavioral, and physical symptoms at these three points in the diet:

- prior to starting the elimination diet
- at the end of the elimination period
- during the challenge phase (when gluten and casein are added back into his diet).

When you add gluten and casein back into your child's diet, I suggest challenging first with casein, then the next week with gluten. This way you can determine if just gluten, just casein, or both are a problem. If your child is a positive responder to the elimination of gluten and/or casein, eliminate them from your child's diet for a year and then re-challenge him. It's possible that he'll no longer have a reaction to gluten and/or casein and will be able to add moderate amounts back into his diet.

An organization called Talking About Curing Autism (TACA) is an excellent resource for parents with autistic kids on the GFCF diet. Visit its Web site at www.talkaboutcuringautism.org.

EXPLORING OTHER ELIMINATION DIETS

The GFCF diet isn't the only elimination diet commonly suggested for autistic children. I don't typically recommend the following diets for autistic children; however, I inform the parents I work with that if they want to try any of these diets, I'll be there to support their decision and help them implement it safely.

The Specific Carbohydrate Diet (SCD)

The Specific Carbohydrate Diet is one of the newer elimination diets and has become quite popular within the autism community over the last few years. It's suggested for treating a small subset of autistic children with gastrointestinal symptoms such as chronic loose stools, intermittent constipation, gas, bloating, and abdominal pain who have been nonresponders to other elimination diets.

The SCD is based on the *theory* that single sugar unit carbohydrates (monosaccharides) are easily digested and well absorbed whereas carbohydrates containing two or more sugar units (disaccharides and polysaccharides) are difficult to digest, especially for those with a compromised gastrointestinal tract and inadequate production of carbohydrate digestive enzymes. If carbohydrates pass undigested through the small intestines into the large intestines, it causes significant intestinal problems. The undigested, unabsorbed carbohydrates that make their way to the large intestines undergo a process called fermentation. Fermentation results in excess gas, bloating, loose stools, constipation, and the production of short-chain organic acids such as lactic and acetic acids, which promotes bacterial overgrowth. Bacterial overgrowth in the intestines leads to intestinal inflammation, which inhibits the absorption of nutrients, especially vitamin B_{12}.

The SCD allows your child to consume the easily digestible single sugar unit monosaccharides (glucose, fructose, and galactose) and eliminates disaccharides (sucrose, lactose, and maltose) and polysaccharides (starches) from his diet. As his gastrointestinal symptoms improve, the disaccharide and polysaccharide carbohydrate foods are gradually added back into his diet as tolerated. The goal of this diet is to correct **dysbiosis** (the imbalance of yeast, bad bacteria, and good bacteria in the gut), decrease intestinal inflammation, heal the intestinal tract, and restore health to the digestive system.

The SCD was originally developed by Dr. Sydney Haas for adults suffering from inflammatory bowel diseases. However, since a large number of autistic children have gastrointestinal symptoms, the diet is now commonly used as a dietary treatment for autism. Many parents of autistic children have tried the SCD and reported positive results in their child's gastrointestinal and behavioral symptoms, increasing its recent popularity in the autism community. If you're interested in trying the SCD, my advice is to proceed with caution. The SCD is a very restrictive diet, making it extremely challenging (even impossible) for many autistic children to follow. Your child must eat a wide variety of foods to be placed on such a restrictive diet. Additionally, in my clinical experience, very few children actually *need* to be on the SCD. I've found that it's usually more beneficial to focus on expanding your child's diet to include adequate protein, healthy fats, unrefined complex carbohydrates, and nutrient-rich simple carbohydrates and limiting excess carbohydrates. This alone is a great start in healing your child's gastrointestinal tract. Before trying such a restrictive diet, I suggest you try the nutritional interventions I've discussed in this book first. You may find that the SCD is not necessary for your child.

The Rotation Diet

The rotation diet is based on the theory that the likelihood your child will have an allergic reaction to a food increases over time with exposure. Many physicians practicing complementary and alternative medicine (CAM) use the IgG ELISA test to identify foods that are believed to cause a delayed food hypersensitivity reaction. These physicians may also use the Mediator Release Test (MRT), which is believed to identify potential non-IgE mediated food reactions. You'll be given a four-day rotation diet plan for your child where a "safe food" is eaten only one day every four days. So on day one, your child can eat all the foods on that day's food list, and these foods will not be eaten again until day four. It's believed that rotating foods every four or more days will minimize reactions and reduce the likelihood of developing an allergy to these foods.

The Antifungal Diet

The antifungal diet, also called a yeast-free diet, is based on the *theory* that autistic children commonly have an overgrowth of **Candida albicans** yeast in their digestive tract, which contributes to "leaky gut syndrome." The antifungal diet is typically used in conjunction with probiotics, antifungals, and medication to get the yeast under control and normalize the microflora balance in the gastrointestinal tract. The diet eliminates foods that contain yeast and foods that supposedly stimulate the growth of yeast. Foods that will be removed from your child's diet include sugar, fruit, fruit juices, fermented foods, baker's yeast, and aged foods. The complete list of foods eliminated on the antifungal diet is quite extensive and includes foods that your child probably eats a lot of. This is another very restrictive diet, so I advise you to proceed with caution and first pursue the nutritional interventions discussed in Step 6 to heal the gastrointestinal tract. More detailed information on the antifungal diet can be found on the Web at www.yeastconnection.com.

The Feingold Diet

The Feingold Diet, also called the Feingold Program, was originally developed by Dr. Ben Feingold in the 1970s. He theorized that certain foods and food additives trigger a variety of adverse physical and behavioral symptoms in sensitive children. Common physical symptoms include headaches, hives, itchy skin, stomach pain, and bed wetting. Behavioral symptoms include hyperactivity and poor concentration. The foods that were believed to be creating these adverse symptoms contained **salicylates**, which are chemicals that occur naturally in many plants. Chemicals used in artificial colors, artificial flavors, preservatives, and aspartame also contain salicylates. The natural salicylate compound found in plants is also chemically similar to manufactured aspirin.

Simply put, the Feingold Diet is a two-stage salicylate elimination diet. In stage one, artificial colors, artificial flavors, preservatives (BHA, BHT, and TBHA), aspartame, foods containing salicylates, and aspirin are eliminated. Foods that contain salicylates include almonds, apples, apricots, berries, cherries, cloves, coffee, cucumbers, currants, grapes, nectarines, oil of wintergreen, oranges, peaches, peppers, pickles, plums, prunes, raisins, tangerines, tea, and tomatoes. After four to six weeks on stage one and symptom improvement is observed in your child, stage two is initiated, which involves adding back foods that contain salicylates. Foods are introduced back into your child's diet one at a time to determine which foods cause an adverse reaction. Some children are hypersensitive to salicylates and may experience significant improvement on the salicylate elimination diet. More often, though, autistic children are sensitive to salicylate-containing chemicals such as artificial colors, artificial flavors, preservatives, and aspartame instead of salicylate-containing foods.

Salicylates are of special interest in the autism community because they may suppress the enzyme **phenol sulfotransferase (PST)**. PST is a key enzyme in the liver responsible for the elimination of toxins from the body. The enormous amount of salicylate-containing chemicals added to our foods put an extra burden on your child's detoxification system. To lessen the burden and enhance your child's detoxification system function, it's best to eliminate artificial colors, artificial flavors, preservatives (BHA, BHT, and TBHA), and aspartame from your child's diet regardless of his reaction to foods containing salicylates.

You can find more detailed information on the Feingold Diet on the Feingold Association of the United States Web site at www.feingold.org.

Vincent's Story

Six-year-old Vincent was nonverbal, had severe tantrums, poor eye contact, avoided interactions with others, and didn't engage with his therapists during therapy sessions. He suffered from loose stools, and his mom told me he had bowel problems since infancy, making it very difficult to start potty training.

Vincent didn't have any significant feeding problems except that he refused to eat fresh fruits and vegetables—he would only eat them cooked. He consumed a variety of foods and accepted new cooked foods after several exposures. An IgE RAST food allergy test indicated he was positive for soy and milk. His mom replaced cow's milk with soy milk, but she allowed him to eat other dairy products. Vincent's mother was very health-conscious, cooked most meals from scratch, and avoided processed and prepackaged foods and artificial colors and flavors.

When I first saw Vincent, his parents were ready to try the GFCF diet. But before we could start the diet, Vincent needed to have completed the steps I describe in this book. His mom had already completed steps 1 through 3; we started Vincent on a omega-3 fatty acid supplement (Step 4); to address his aversion to fresh fruits and vegetables, he started feeding therapy with his current therapists (Step 5); since he had a history of gastrointestinal problems, we started a gut healing program of digestive enzymes and probiotics (Step 6), which significantly improved his loose stools but didn't completely normalize them; and since allergy testing indicated that he may be allergic to cow's milk and soy, we combined steps 7 and 8, eliminating soy along with gluten and casein.

Before Vincent began the GFCF diet, his parents, therapists, and teacher documented his current symptoms to obtain a baseline for comparison. Since Vincent didn't have any serious feeding problems, he easily transitioned to a gluten-, casein-, and soy-free diet within a few weeks. His parents, therapists, and teacher continued to record his symptoms on a weekly basis to document his response to the diet. After two weeks or so without gluten, casein, and soy, they began to note improvements in Vincent. His behavior improved, he had fewer tantrums, a higher tolerance level to frustration, and better eye contact. His mom noted that his bowel problem was totally resolved; he had normally formed stools for the first time and was able to start potty training. As the weeks went by over the three-month period, they saw continued improvement in his behavior, and he became more engaged with his siblings and other people in his environment. The therapists were very excited about Vincent's new willingness to cooperate and interact during the speech and occupational therapy sessions. Everyone commented that Vincent was smiling, appeared happier, and was just a pleasant child. At the end of the three-month elimination phase, everyone agreed that the GFCF diet was helping Vincent and should be continued.

Now it was time to challenge Vincent and determine which food protein was contributing to which symptoms. The first week soy was added back into Vincent's diet. His parents, therapists, and teacher watched for regression in any of his behavioral or gastrointestinal symptoms but saw none, so soy was allowed back into his diet. The second week, cow's milk and other dairy products were added back into his diet. Within a few days his mom noted that Vincent had a return of loose stools; so cow's milk and all dairy products were eliminated from his diet. The third week gluten was added back, and within one day his therapists and teacher observed slight regression in his behavior. A few days later they reported that Vincent continued to regress to the point where he was having daily tantrums, was uncooperative in therapy sessions, and was functioning at the level prior to starting the GFCF diet. Since Vincent's regression was so significant, the gluten challenge was immediately stopped. After a few days back on the GFCF diet Vincent's behavioral symptoms improved, reinforcing that he was a positive responder to the diet.

The school staff who were involved in observing Vincent's response to the GFCF diet were so impressed with the benefits that they asked if they could add nutrition goals, objectives, and support services to Vincent's Individual Education Program (IEP). His IEP team agreed that Vincent wouldn't benefit from his special education services unless he was on the GFCF diet, so it was an educational need. This meant that Special Education funds could be allocated to purchase gluten- and casein-free foods for Vincent's school lunch and pay a consulting registered dietitian to review the school menus and recommend modifications.

PROJECT NO. 8: IS YOUR CHILD A POSITIVE RESPONDER TO THE GFCF DIET?

1. Talk to a knowledgeable registered dietitian who can help you implement the GFCF diet.

2. Conduct a three-month elimination of gluten, casein, and soy, making sure to document your child's symptoms prior to and at the end of the elimination phase. List any specific symptom improvements.

3. Challenge with soy first, then casein, then gluten to determine if symptoms return.

4. If your child is a positive responder, continue to eliminate gluten, casein, and/or soy from his diet.

Although they're not recommended by most medical professionals, special elimination diets continue to be very popular in the autism community. Until more science-based research is available, parents will have to conduct a "mini-experiment" on their own children to determine if the elimination of certain foods is beneficial to them. I've had a lot of success with the GFCF diet and think it's worth your taking some time to consider trying it.

Now it's time to move on to Step 9, which involves another controversial yet popular nutritional treatment in the autism community—treating your child's symptoms with a very high dosage of vitamin B_6.

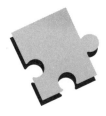

STEP 9

Try High Dose Vitamin B₆ with Magnesium

People typically supplement their diet with vitamins as a way to ward off disease and prevent vitamin deficiencies. The goal for using high-dose vitamins is completely different. A high-dose vitamin regimen, also known as "megavitamin therapy" and "orthomolecular medicine," involves taking large amounts of a single, specific vitamin to achieve a particular health benefit. For instance, high doses of niacin are used to treat mental disorders such as schizophrenia and hypercholesterolemia, and high doses of vitamin C are used to treat cancer and AIDS. In the autism community, a high dose of vitamin B_6 coupled with magnesium is the treatment of interest.

It's important to point out that while complementary and alternative medicine (CAM) practitioners frequently use megavitamin therapy to treat a wide range of conditions, the mainstream medical community considers the practice poorly supported by scientific research, ineffective, and potentially harmful and doesn't support it.

MEGAVITAMIN THERAPY AND AUTISM

The use of megavitamin therapy gained popularity in the autism community in the 1960s, when the idea that daily high doses of vitamin B_6 (pyridoxine) may benefit autistic children was introduced. Today, high dose vitamin B_6 is the most popular megavitamin therapy used to treat the condition. Here's a list of beneficial effects autistic children have reportedly experienced:

- behavioral improvement
- decreased aggression
- fewer tantrums

- improved social responsiveness
- less stimulatory behavior
- increased speech
- improved eye contact

There have been more than a dozen research studies done on high dose vitamin B_6 treatment for autism, and many of them concluded that it benefits up to half of autistic children. However, only a few of these research studies were double-blind, randomized, placebo-controlled trials, and many medical professionals believe that the studies were poorly designed, biased, or had inadequate sample sizes. Additionally, the doses of vitamin B_6 used in these research studies varied greatly, so it's still not clear what the appropriate dosage to treat autism should be.

A key finding of these research studies was that high doses of vitamin B_6 were effective for improving autistic symptoms only when used in combination with magnesium. Magnesium is a mineral involved in more than three hundred biochemical reactions in the body. It helps maintain normal nerve function, supports a healthy immune system, helps to regulate blood glucose levels, is involved in the synthesis of protein and energy production, and helps regulate blood pressure.

Overall, the results of these studies suggest that high dose vitamin B_6 with magnesium may well be effective in improving certain characteristics of autism.

WHY VITAMIN B_6?

The autism community has focused on vitamin B_6 as an avenue of treatment because of the role it plays in neurological function. Vitamin B_6 is a water-soluble vitamin that's essential to the synthesis of serotonin and dopamine, two key neurotransmitters in the brain.

Serotonin plays an important role in the modulation of mood, anger, aggression, sleep, and appetite. Low levels of serotonin are associated with a susceptibility to depression, anxiety, aggression, and **obsessive-compulsive disorder (OCD)**.

Dopamine plays an important role in mood, sleep, motor activity, and behavior. It's critical for cognitive functions such as attention, learning, memory, and problem solving. Dopamine is also involved in motivation and reward by signaling parts of the brain responsible for learning to repeat behaviors that lead to reward. Low levels of dopamine have been associated with autism, ADHD, schizophrenia, and social anxiety.

In essence, high dose vitamin B_6 is being used as a "medication" to naturally increase the production of serotonin and dopamine in the brain. This neurological connection may explain why it's been effective in improving symptoms for some autistic children. Vitamin B$_6$ plays many roles within the body. It helps with the following:

- creating neurotransmitters such as serotonin and dopamine

- forming and maintaining the central nervous system

- aiding more than one hundred enzymes in the metabolism of protein

- helping the immune system function properly

- creating hemoglobin

- maintaining blood glucose levels within a normal range

- maintaining the health of lymphoid organs, such as the tonsils, adenoids, lymph nodes, and spleen

DETERMINING THE RIGHT VITAMIN B$_6$ DOSAGE FOR YOUR CHILD

Unfortunately, there's no clear-cut dosage to which autistic children seem to respond. The amounts of B$_6$ used in the research studies I discussed earlier varied greatly. Theoretically, since we are all biochemically unique, some autistic children may require a higher dosage than others. This can be confusing when you're trying to figure out the right amount of B$_6$ to use for your child.

Typically, the amount of vitamin B$_6$ that health practitioners suggest using exceeds both the RDA and the UL recommended by the USDA Food and Nutrition Board. B$_6$ dosages can range from 200, 500, to even 1,000 mg per day. Many practitioners follow the guidelines set forth by the Autism Research Institute (ARI), which bases its suggestions on informal data collection from parents of autistic children (see www.autism.com for more information). According to the ARI, the average amount of vitamin B$_6$ found to be beneficial is 8 mg per pound of body weight per day. For example, a 35-pound child would take 280 mg of vitamin B$_6$ per day. Here are some additional ARI guidelines to follow as you start your child on a high dose B$_6$ regimen:

- Start at one quarter the total dosage and increase to the full dosage over a fourteen-day period of time.

- If the high dose vitamin B$_6$ is effective, you should see the benefits within a few days.

• If you don't see any improvements within a month, the high dose vitamin B_6 should be stopped.

You also need to make sure your child is taking in an adequate amount of magnesium along with the vitamin B_6. The ARI suggests taking 3 to 4 mg of magnesium per pound of body weight per day up to a maximum of 400 mg per day in adults. For example, a 35-pound child would take 105 to 140 mg of magnesium per day in addition to his high dose B_6.

PYRIDOXINE AND PYRIDOXAL 5-PHOSPHATE (P5P) ARE NOT THE SAME THING

Please be careful not to confuse pyridoxine, also known as vitamin B_6, with Pyridoxal 5-phosphate (P5P). P5P is the active form of pyridoxine—the body has to convert pyridoxine to P5P in order to use it, and this conversion is dependent upon the minerals magnesium and zinc. Some healthcare practitioners believe that autistic children may have difficulty converting pyridoxine to P5P, so they suggest using supplemental P5P or a combination of pyridoxine and P5P supplements. The supposed advantages are that an autistic child wouldn't need to convert pyridoxine to P5P because he's taking it in its active form, and its effectiveness wouldn't be compromised if he has a magnesium or zinc deficiency. We know that supplemental P5P should be taken at a lower dosage than pyridoxine, but no controlled studies have yielded an exact recommendation for how much P5P should be used to replace pyridoxine. If you choose to do a trial response for high dose vitamin B_6, I recommend you use B_6 in the form of pyridoxine, not P5P.

CONCERNS ABOUT SAFETY

The major concern about taking any vitamin at a high dose is the potential for toxicity. When vitamin B_6 is consumed through food sources, there are no adverse effects. However, when taken in supplement form in high doses, toxicity can become an issue. There are no problems associated with short-term use, but when taken at high levels for months or years, it may cause problems like **sensory neuropathy**, a condition characterized by numbness, tingling, and burning pain commonly in the hands, arms, feet, and legs. The adverse effects are reversible if the symptoms are identified and the high dose vitamin B_6 supplementation is immediately stopped.

Recognizing Adverse Effects

It's highly unlikely that your child will develop a side effect such as sensory neuropathy. Still, you should learn to recognize the signs of a problem should it occur, especially if your child is nonverbal. If your child demonstrates any of the following symptoms, take him off the high dose B$_6$ immediately:

• shakes his hands

• wrenches his hands

• increases hand stimming

• walks on his tiptoes

Diarrhea is a potential side effect of taking excessive magnesium in supplement form, so many practitioners suggest limiting the amount of magnesium in supplements to the UL. Here's an at-a-glance table with the UL for supplemental magnesium:

Age	UL Magnesium (mg/day)
1–3 years	65
4–8 years	110
8 years and older	350

Based on 5mg per kilogram of body weight per day.

Source: USDA. Food and Nutrition Board, National Academy of Sciences, Institute of Medicine

DECIDING IF HIGH DOSE VITAMIN B$_6$ IS RIGHT FOR YOUR CHILD

There's no test to determine if your child will benefit from high dose vitamin B$_6$. The only way to know if it will benefit your child is to try it. If you do decide to move forward, I strongly encourage you to enlist the help of a registered dietitian or nutrition-oriented physician before starting. Discussing the pros and cons of a high dose vitamin B$_6$ regimen with the appropriate medical professional is the best way to make a fully informed decision for your child. The medical professional can also help you select an appropriate product, proper dosage, conduct a safe trial response, determine if B$_6$ is effective or not, and decide if the high dose vitamin B$_6$ should be continued or not.

There's great debate over the effectiveness of high dose vitamin B_6 with magnesium to treat autism among healthcare practitioners. Organizations such as the Autism Research Institute (ARI) and physicians practicing complementary and alternative medicine advocate for its use, but very few conventional physicians and even fewer registered dietitians support it. Since a growing number of parents are using high dose vitamin B_6 to treat their child's autistic symptoms, this means that many of them are doing so without the approval of their physician or help from a registered dietitian. I firmly believe that if a parent chooses to try their child on high dose vitamin B_6, they should not be left to go through the process alone. If you find yourself in this position, I urge you to find a doctor and/or dietitian who will support your decision, so you can safely conduct a trial response for your child with medical supervision.

CONDUCTING A TRIAL RESPONSE

When I work with parents who want to try their child on high dose vitamin B_6, I have them conduct a one-month trial response to determine whether their child is a positive responder. A trial response is basically a "mini-experiment" designed to gather objective information so you can make an informed decision about whether your child benefits from high dose vitamin B_6. This means it's very important that you remain objective, systematic, and observant and document all results.

Here's the procedure:

1. Choose a medical professional to help you.

2. With the medical professional, select a high dose vitamin B_6 supplement product.

3. Jointly decide on the full dosage of vitamin B_6 per day, the amount to initially start with, and how much to increase weekly to reach the full dosage.

4. Make sure your child is consuming at least the RDA for magnesium in a supplement.

5. You and your child's caregivers, therapists, and teachers should document his symptoms prior to starting the high dose vitamin B_6 (known as baseline data). Current symptoms to document should include your child's communication skills, social interaction, behavior, stereotyped activities, sleep, bed wetting, hyperactivity, focus, attention, feeding problems, and bowel function.

6. Begin the high dose vitamin B$_6$.

7. You and your child's caregivers, therapists, and teachers should document his symptoms on a weekly basis. This is known as response data, and it's important because many autistic children have a positive response to B$_6$ at a lower dosage and don't require the full dosage.

8. Gradually increase your child's dosage weekly until you reach the full dosage; continue the trial response for approximately two more weeks once the full dosage is reached.

9. You and your child's caregivers, therapists, and teachers should separately evaluate your documented observations (evaluation data) and determine if the high dose was beneficial for your child.

10. You and the medical professional you're working with should assess all the data collected on your child and decide whether the high dose vitamin B$_6$ should be continued. See Appendix 5 for examples of baseline, response, and evaluation forms that you can use to document your child's symptoms and response.

If, after comparing all the data, you conclude that the high dose vitamin B$_6$ had no beneficial effects or actually made your child's symptoms worse, take him off it.

If you determine that the high dose vitamin B$_6$ resulted in substantial improvement and/or improvement in one or more of your child's symptoms, it may be beneficial for him and you may want to continue the regimen.

If you conclude that the vitamin B$_6$ resulted in a combination of positive and negative results, discuss with your medical professional and decide whether or not high dose vitamin B$_6$ should be continued.

If you decide your child should continue the high dose vitamin B$_6$, I suggest you have him reassessed after six months. The truth is that it's impossible to be 100 percent sure your child is a positive responder because of all the other therapies he may be undergoing at the same time he began his B$_6$ regimen. At the six-month mark you should conduct a second trial response, which involves stopping the high dose vitamin B$_6$ and watching for the return of any of your child's symptoms. If you don't see any symptom regression, then the high dose vitamin B$_6$ may not be beneficial after all and can be discontinued. On the other hand, if his symptoms do regress, then the high dose vitamin B$_6$ is likely beneficial and should be continued. If you decide to continue the high dose vitamin B$_6$ beyond six months, be sure to tell your child's doctor that he's on a thera-peutic level of vitamin B$_6$ and watch for signs of sensory neuropathy.

Many autistic children take Super Nu Thera, which is a daily multivitamin and min-eral supplement that also contains a high dose of vitamin B$_6$. It's available in caplets, powder, and liquid form and with or without vitamins A and D. Please note that if you try Super Nu Thera and your child's one month trial response indicates that vitamin B$_6$ isn't beneficial to him, you'll need to replace the Super Nu Thera with a basic multivit-amin and mineral supplement. Super Nu Thera is distributed by Kirkman, and you can visit www.kirkmangroup.com for information on this product.

Maria's Story

Maria is a good example of a patient of mine who had a positive response to high dose vitamin B$_6$. Maria was four years old and diagnosed with autism. She was considered high functioning and received therapy through an Early Childhood Program at her local public school. Her mother told me that Maria was easily frustrated, flapped her arms when overwhelmed, retreated into her own world, avoided eye contact, and had delayed speech.

Based on Maria's body weight of 32 pounds, the suggested high dose vitamin B$_6$ dosage was approximately 250 mg per day (8 mg vitamin B$_6$ per pound of body weight). The suggested magnesium dose was approximately 96–128 mg per day (3–4 mg magnesium per pound of body weight). Maria's parents purchased vitamin B$_6$ in 50 mg pull-apart capsules so the powder could be mixed into soft food. Her daily multivitamin and mineral supplement contained an adequate amount of magnesium, so a magnesium supplement wasn't necessary. Before starting the one-month trial response of high dose vitamin B$_6$, Maria's parents, teacher, and therapists completed the Baseline Data form on page 234 to document her existing symptoms. The high dose vitamin B$_6$ was started at 50 mg per day, and increased by 50 mg increments every two or three days until the full dosage of 250 mg was reached in two weeks. The Response Data form was completed at the end of each week to monitor her progress. At the end of the one-month trial response, the Evaluation Data form was filled out to assess whether the high dose vitamin B$_6$ was beneficial. Everyone agreed that Maria had notable improvement in eye contact, wasn't as easily frustrated, and demonstrated less arm flapping after starting the high dose vitamin B$_6$, so it was continued. Six months later, Maria underwent another trial response. This time the high dose vitamin B$_6$ was gradually decreased in 50 mg increments over two weeks, to determine if Maria's symptoms would regress without the high dose vitamin B$_6$. Maria's parents, teacher, and therapists again observed, documented her symptoms, and noted that Maria did regress when the high dose vitamin B$_6$ was decreased. Maria's parents felt the high dose vitamin B$_6$ was beneficial, chose to continue it, and informed Maria's physician of their decision.

PROJECT NO. 9: IS YOUR CHILD A POSITIVE RESPONDER TO HIGH DOSE VITAMIN B$_6$?

1. With the help of a medical professional, calculate the proper vitamin B$_6$ dosage for your child and choose a product (either Super Nu Thera or a simple B$_6$ supplement).

2. Calculate the proper dosage of magnesium that should accompany the B$_6$.

3. Record your child's baseline symptoms (see form in Appendix 5).

4. Initiate the trial response and document his response data (see form in Appendix 5).

5. At the end of one month, evaluate all the data you've collected and see if he's shown any symptom improvement. If so, your child is a positive responder to a high dose vitamin B$_6$ regimen.

High dose vitamin B$_6$ isn't the only nutrient used in advanced nutritional interventions to treat autism. Many other vitamins, minerals, herbs, amino acids, and nutraceuticals are also suggested for autistic children, and we tackle those in the final step of this program.

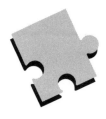

STEP 10

Explore Additional Supplements

There are many other vitamins, minerals, antioxidants, amino acids, nutraceuticals, and herbs believed to benefit autistic children. These supplements are accepted and commonly used as advanced nutritional treatment in the autism community.

Before we get started, it's important to understand that each of these advanced nutritional supplementations serves a very specific purpose, and not every autistic child needs them. Some autistic children will use most of them, other children only a few supplements, and still others should not try any advanced supplements because they aren't appropriate for their individual conditions. Also, contrary to what many medical practitioners tell parents, you should *not* start your child on all of these supplements at once, nor should they all be used at the same time. Many parents end up purchasing dozens of expensive supplements and try to get their child to take all of these supplements every day, which never works. Doing so will only make you feel frustrated, overwhelmed, and totally disillusioned with all nutritional interventions. Treating autism is like running a marathon—you need to start slowly and pace yourself. Work with your child's registered dietitian or nutrition-oriented physician to figure out which advanced supplements, if any, might be appropriate for your child. Lastly, do not even attempt to implement this step until your child has mastered the first nine steps of my program. His basic nutrition must be in place before you delve into more advanced interventions.

ADVANCED SUPPLEMENTS

Since there are so many advanced supplements to consider, it's easiest to group them together by their intended purpose. Some supplements are used to enhance the detoxification or immune systems, some to enhance cognitive function, and others to improve behavioral or other autistic symptoms. You'll quickly see which groups of supplements may be appropriate to treat your child's individual symptoms. Please note that the groupings are not all-inclusive but rather a general guideline to help you start a discussion with your child's registered dietitian or physician. A few of these supplements are considered controversial and are not recommended by some medical professionals. You'll need to work with someone who's willing to have open discussions about all of these supplements so you can make a well-informed decision regarding their use for your child.

Supplements to Enhance Cognitive Function

The following supplements are used because of their ability to enhance a child's comprehension, reasoning, decision making, planning, and learning abilities:

- carnitine
- choline
- coenzyme Q_{10} (CoQ_{10})
- iron
- zinc

Carnitine

Carnitine is the generic term for the compounds L-carnitine, acetyl-L-carnitine, and propionyl-L-carnitine. It's synthesized in the body from the essential amino acids lysine and methionine. Carnitine plays a critical role in energy production, transporting long-chain fatty acids into the mitochondria so they can be burned to produce energy. It then transports waste out of the cell to prevent waste accumulation. Carnitine may also have brain and central nervous system protection abilities, cardio protective activity, triglyceride-lowering effects, and antioxidant properties. One research study has suggested that 50 percent of boys with ADD have a positive response to L-carnitine supplements.

A deficiency in carnitine can cause your child to have muscle weakness, **hypoglycemia**, and elevated blood-ammonia concentrations. Carnitine deficiencies can be caused by valproic acid, which is a medication used to treat seizures, as well as some antibiotics. There's also a genetic disorder called **primary carnitine deficiency**, which manifests by five years of age, in which a child's carnitine transporters don't work properly. I recommend that you ask your child's physician to order a carnitine blood test to determine if he has a deficiency and needs supplementation. The following are carnitine-rich foods:

meat (the redder the meat, the higher
   the carnitine content)

fish

poultry

milk

dairy products
   (in the whey component)

To determine if your child may benefit from carnitine supplementation, you should do a trial response under the supervision of his doctor. (See page 124 in Step 9 for a refresher on how to conduct a trial response. You'll find trial response forms in Appendix 5 that you can use to document your child's symptoms and response to carnitine.) Be on the lookout for symptoms of excess carnitine, such as nausea, vomiting, abdominal cramps, and diarrhea. Carnitine is available by prescription under the brand name Carnitor and the generic levocarnitine and over-the-counter in the form of L-carnitine and acetyl-L-carnitine. There is currently no RDA for carnitine. For dosage recommendations for over-the-counter carnitine, refer to the PDR for Nutritional Supplements.

Choline

Choline is a water-soluble nutrient that the body needs to make several important compounds necessary for healthy cell membranes. It's a component of phosphatidylcholine (lecithin) and the neurotransmitter acetylcholine, which is one of the crucial brain chemicals involved in memory. Choline is also a precursor for the methyl donor trimethylglycine (TMG). A few reports indicate that choline can improve short-term memory skills and enhance memory in poor learners. The Food and Nutrition Board of the National Academy of Sciences recommends that pregnant and nursing women increase their intake of choline to help ensure normal fetal brain development. The American Academy of Pediatrics (AAP) recommends that infant formula contain choline. There's currently no RDA for choline, but the Food and Nutrition Board of the Institute of Medicine of the National Academy of Sciences has established Adequate Intakes, which are listed in Appendix 3. The following are choline-rich foods:

organ meats	pork	nuts
egg yolks	fish	beans
beef	poultry	peanut butter
soy protein powder	cauliflower	Brussels sprouts

Too much supplemental choline has been reported to cause nausea, diarrhea, and loose stools. Supplemental choline comes in several different forms, and I recommend that you stay away from choline in the form of choline bitartrate. There are indications that it may increase symptoms of depression.

Coenzyme Q$_{10}$

Coenzyme Q$_{10}$ is a fat-soluble substance that belongs to a family of substances called **ubiquinones**. CoQ$_{10}$ has antioxidant properties that protect the central nervous system and the brain from neurodegenerative diseases. Since CoQ$_{10}$ is recognized as such an important antioxidant for the brain, it's commonly added to daily multivitamin and mineral supplements. Check your child's daily supplement to see if he's already getting CoQ$_{10}$. If so, an additional supplement isn't necessary. If you do decide to try your child on a CoQ$_{10}$ supplement, discuss dosage with your child's registered dietitian or physician, as there's no RDA for CoQ$_{10}$. For dosage recommendations, I refer to the PDR for Nutritional Supplements. Excess amounts of CoQ$_{10}$ can cause your child to experience mild gastrointestinal symptoms such as nausea, diarrhea, and indigestion. The following are CoQ$_{10}$-rich foods:

meat	fish	nuts
poultry	soybean oil	canola oil

Iron

Iron is an essential trace mineral that's critical to your child's brain function. It transports oxygen to cells throughout the body, helps produce carnitine, and is involved in the production of the neurotransmitters serotonin, dopamine, and norepinephrine. Iron is also important to your child's immune function, increasing his resistance to disease and infections. If your child is suffering from an iron deficiency, it can prevent his brain cells from getting the proper amount of oxygen, which can result in compromised mental function, apathy, short attention span, irritability, decreased ability to learn, and impaired school performance. He may also be more vulnerable to Candida, viruses, and other pathogens. There are several routine blood tests, such as the **serum ferritin**, **total iron binding capacity**, hemoglobin and hematocrit tests, that can identify whether your child has even a mild case of iron deficiency anemia. Research studies show that when children with iron deficiency anemia take an iron supplement, their cognitive skills improve and their learning problems diminish.

Since iron is so critical to your child's health, it should already be included in his daily diet through food or a multivitamin and mineral supplement. The following are iron-rich foods:

organ meats	beans	tofu
red meat	soybeans	spinach
fish	lentils	peas
poultry	blackstrap molasses	raisins

If your child doesn't have an iron deficiency and is already getting 100 percent of his RDA for iron, I don't suggest giving him an additional supplement. If too much iron builds up in the body, it can lead to the formation of harmful free radicals that damage cells and contribute to cancer. If tests show your child does suffer from an iron deficiency and requires iron supplementation beyond his RDA, a physician should prescribe it.

Taking too much iron at one time is toxic and can have serious consequences, such as the following:

vomiting	renal failure	lethargy
diarrhea	shock	hypoglycemia
central nervous system depression	coma	liver damage

It's extremely important to keep iron supplements in a childproof bottle and away from children. You can find your child's RDA and Tolerable Upper Intake Level (UL) for iron in Appendix 3.

Zinc

Zinc is an essential mineral involved in the activity of more than one hundred enzymes in the body. Perhaps most importantly, zinc is required for the development and activation of T-lymphocytes, which are the white blood cells that fight infection. Like iron, it's important for your child's growth and development and should already be included in his daily diet through food or a multivitamin and mineral supplement. A zinc deficiency can result in immune dysfunction, growth retardation, loss of appetite, diarrhea, and mental lethargy. Even a moderate zinc deficiency will negatively affect your child's immune system. (Too much zinc will also impair your child's immune function.) The following is a list of zinc-rich foods:

oysters and some other types of seafood	beans	poultry
fortified breakfast cereals	nuts	dairy products
red meat	whole grains	

You can find your child's RDA and UL for zinc in Appendix 3.

SUPPLEMENTS TO ENHANCE THE IMMUNE SYSTEM

- Dimethylglycine (DMG)
- Iron
- Magnesium
- Selenium
- Vitamin A
- Vitamin C
- Vitamin D
- Vitamin E
- Zinc

By now you know that many medical professionals within the autism community believe that autistic children are more prone to immune system dysfunction than other children. Physicians who treat autism with alternative and complementary interventions often recommend controversial treatments such as **intravenous immune globulin (IVIG), oral immunoglobulin (OIG), transfer factors,** and antiviral, antifungal, and antibacterial medications. Many parents prefer to play it safe by sticking with vitamins, minerals, and nutrients that naturally enhance their child's immune system. Your child's registered dietitian can help you ensure he's getting enough iron, magnesium, selenium, zinc, and vitamins A, C, D, and E through food and/or a daily multivitamin and mineral supplement. Your child should be taking in at least his RDA but should not exceed his UL.

Dimethylglycine (DMG)

Dimethylglycine is a water-soluble substance found naturally in animal and plant cells. Animal research indicates that DMG may support the immune system. Some foods that are rich in dimethlyglycine are beans, cereal grain, and liver. The PDR for Nutritional Supplements suggest the typical dose is 125 mg per day. DMG is nontoxic, and no adverse reactions have been reported.

In the autism community, many have reported that DMG can improve an autistic child's behavior, eye contact, and expressive language. Unfortunately, the three small research studies that have been conducted on DMG and autism don't support this. Still, parents continue to try DMG with their autistic children, and it remains one of the most popular supplements. If you are interested in trying DMG to enhance your child's expressive language, you can check the Autism Research Institute Web site for dosage suggestions for your child. I encourage you to first talk with his registered dietitian or physician before starting a trial response to determine if he's a positive responder to DMG.

David's Story

Five-year-old David was diagnosed with autism. He made little eye contact, repeated words in place of normal language, lined up toys, had numerous tantrums and behavioral problems, was easily frustrated, and had difficulty falling and staying asleep at night. David's mother said he had developmental delays since birth. He'd had frequent ear infections as an infant that were treated with numerous rounds of antibiotics. He suffered with loose stools, was gaseous, and never had normal formed bowel movements. He also had a history of frequent illnesses such as colds, bronchitis, and pneumonia. David refused to eat any fruits or vegetables and consumed a very limited variety of foods. An IgE RAST allergy test indicated that he was allergic to egg white, but eggs hadn't been eliminated from his diet. The only supplement David was taking was a liquid baby vitamin supplement. David's parents had not tried any nutritional interventions or dietary changes before consulting with me.

I had the opportunity to work with David over several months and help his parents implement the entire 10-Step Nutrition Plan. His parents were eager to get started and quickly completed steps 1 and 2. The entire family transitioned to consuming healthier, whole, organic foods and avoided foods with trans fat, excess sugar, and refined carbohydrates. David's parents made sure he was consuming adequate protein, healthy fats, complex carbohydrates, and filtered water on a daily basis. Step 3 and 4 were quickly and easily achieved by replacing the liquid baby vitamin supplement with a children's daily multivitamin and mineral supplement and starting David on an omega-3 fatty acid supplement. To address his refusal of fruits and vegetables and his limited food repertoire, David began feeding therapy at a private out-patient feeding clinic (Step 5). Since he had gastrointestinal problems, we initiated the gut healing program (Step 6) using probiotics, digestive enzymes, and antifungals, which resolved his runny, loose stools. We knew that David might be allergic to egg white, so we conducted an elimination/challenge diet (Step 7) to determine if he had any negative reactions. He didn't, so eggs were allowed to remain in his diet. Then we began to transition David to the GFCF diet (Step 8). Soon he no longer had sleep problems and his excess gas and bowel problems were resolved, so the GFCF diet was continued. David's parents were interested in how David would respond to high dose vitamin B_6 (Step 9), so we conducted a one-month trial response. It was determined that David was not a positive responder, and the high dose vitamin B$_6$ was discontinued. After completing steps 1 through 9, David had significant improvements in his bowel function, sleep, behavior, feeding problem, and overall autistic symptoms.

David's parents wanted to begin Step 10 and address some of the individual issues impacting David. We first considered trying additional nutritional supplements to enhance his immune system, since he had a history of frequent illness. David's frequent illnesses were a serious concern for his parents because during the winter months David was always sick, missed an extensive number of days from school, and regressed academically. He also missed out on critical speech and occupational therapy sessions, which slowed down his progress. I assessed David's diet and vitamin and mineral supplement to make sure he was getting at least 100 percent of his RDA for the nutrients critical for immune function—iron, magnesium, selenium, zinc and vitamins A, D, and E. I also suggested an additional supplement of 200 mg vitamin C and 125 mg dimethylglycine (DMG) to support the immune system. David's mother reported that this was the first winter during which he didn't suffer from any colds or bronchitis and wasn't hospitalized for pneumonia. She was thrilled that David was able to get through the entire winter without getting sick, being absent from school, and missing speech and occupational therapy sessions.

Magnesium

Magnesium plays a role in more than three hundred biochemical reactions in the body. Its numerous functions include supporting the immune system, helping to build bones, regulating blood sugar levels, protein synthesis, energy metabolism, maintaining normal nerve function, and regulating heart rhythm. If your child isn't getting enough magnesium, he may experience a loss of appetite, confusion, diarrhea, nausea, fatigue, and muscle weakness. Here are some magnesium-rich foods:

halibut	beans	banana	milk
nuts	peas	avocado	
seeds	whole unrefined grains		

Taking too much magnesium in supplement form often causes diarrhea, nausea, and abdominal cramping. Appendix 3 shows your child's RDA and UL for magnesium.

Selenium

Selenium is a trace mineral that the body requires only in very small amounts. Its most important role is as an antioxidant that helps prevent cellular damage caused by free radicals. Selenium also helps support the immune system, regulate thyroid function, protect against some cancers, and rid the body of heavy metals by forming an inactive complex with these metals. If your child suffers from a selenium deficiency, it can weaken his immune system, cause hypothyroidism, spur the development of heart disease, and increase his risk of some cancers. If your child has a gastrointestinal problem such as chronic diarrhea and inflammation, he has an increased risk for selenium deficiency because his body is less able to absorb it. The following are selenium-rich foods:

brazil nuts	cod	eggs	enriched bread
tuna	turkey	oatmeal	
beef	chicken	rice	

Taking too much selenium can result in **selenosis**, the symptoms of which include irritability, fatigue, nausea, vomiting, garliclike breath, hair loss, and white, blotchy nails. See Appendix 3 for your child's RDA and UL for selenium.

Vitamin A

Vitamin A is actually a group of fat-soluble substances. **Preformed vitamin A**, or vitamin A that occurs in a form ready to be used by the body, is found in animal sources. **Carotenoids** are found in plant sources and must be converted to vitamin A. (You've probably heard of beta carotene, which is the most common carotenoid.) Vitamin A is critical to the proper functioning of the immune system. It's involved in making white blood cells, which destroy harmful bacteria and viruses. Vitamin A also plays a major role in vision, brain development, growth, and bone development, and its antioxidant properties may help prevent cancer. If your child has a vitamin A deficiency, it will compromise his immune system and make him susceptible to many types of infection. Even a mild deficiency can cause a loss of appetite, decreased growth rate, slow bone development, and night blindness. Some foods that are rich in preformed vitamin A are:

liver	egg yolk	cream	whole milk
fish liver oils	butter	fortified skim milk	

Here are some carotenoid-rich foods:

carrots	kale	apricots	mango	peas	tomatoes
spinach	cantaloupe	papaya	peaches	red pepper	

Too much vitamin A can result in **hypervitaminosis A**, a condition where high levels of the vitamin are stored within the body. This excess of vitamin A can be toxic and cause reactions such as nausea, vomiting, headache, muscular uncoordination, reduced bone density, liver damage, and birth defects. Hypervitaminosis A typically occurs only when taking preformed vitamin A supplements. Turn to Appendix 3 to find your child's RDA and UL for vitamin A.

Vitamin C

Vitamin C is a water-soluble vitamin that performs a variety of important functions. It helps support the immune system; in fact, several research studies indicate that vitamin C decreases the incidence, duration, and severity of the common cold. Its antioxidant properties help prevent chronic diseases such as cancer, heart disease, and cataracts caused by oxidative damage. Vitamin C increases the body's ability to absorb iron, heal wounds, and protects against asthma. Vitamin C is a cofactor in the carnitine transport system and the conversion of tryptophan to serotonin, and it preserves intracellular glutathione concentrations. It also plays a major role in the detoxification system, helping the body get rid of pesticides and heavy metals. Research indicates that high serum levels of ascorbic acid (the major dietary form of vitamin C) are associated with a decreased incidence of high blood lead levels. One research study indicated that ascorbic acid had chelating properties comparable to EDTA, a lead-chelating agent, and is equally able to lower blood-lead levels. (See the section about Chelation Therapy on page 140 for more on this topic).

If your child is vitamin C deficient, his wounds may not heal as quickly, he may have a lower resistance to colds and infections, and he may be more susceptible to a variety of chronic diseases. In severe instances, scurvy can occur, which causes bleeding gums, loosened teeth, muscle weakness, fatigue, loss of appetite, diarrhea, pulmonary problems, and kidney problems. Here are some vitamin C–rich foods:

orange juice	tomato juice	oranges	cantaloupe
Brussels sprouts	cabbage	broccoli	kiwi
strawberries	asparagus	collard greens	
green peas	potatoes	pineapple	

Since excess vitamin C is excreted in the urine, your child can consume large amounts without risk to his health. However, large doses for an extended period of time sometimes result in problems such as nausea, vomiting, stomach cramps, and diarrhea. You can find your child's RDA and UL for vitamin C in Appendix 3. For suggested dosages to enhance the immune and detoxification systems, his dietitian may refer to the PDR for Nutritional Supplements.

In the autism community, vitamin C gained attention because emerging research showed that megadoses of vitamin C had a positive effect on the behavior of autistic children. If you are interested in conducting a trial response of high dose vitamin C to see if your child is a positive responder, be sure to discuss dosage with your child's registered dietitian or physician.

Vitamin D

Vitamin D is a fat-soluble vitamin that aids in the absorption of calcium and phosphorus, helping to form and maintain strong bones and teeth. Vitamin D supports the immune system by boosting **natural killer cells**. Recent research suggests vitamin D may provide protection from certain cancers, type I and type II diabetes, glucose intolerance, high blood pressure, cochlear deafness, and multiple sclerosis. There's also speculation that it plays a role in modulating mood by affecting serotonin levels in the brain. In children, vitamin D deficiency causes rickets, which results in skeletal deformities, soft bones, muscle weakness, and delayed development of teeth. Deficiencies are most often found in children who follow a milk-free or strict vegetarian diet. Some foods that are rich in vitamin D are (note: Vitamin D is also produced by our bodies when our skin is exposed to sunlight):

cod liver oil	sardines	eggs
salmon	fortified milk	liver
mackerel	fortified margarine	cheese
tuna fish	ready-to-eat cereals	

Too much vitamin D can result in symptoms such as nausea, vomiting, weakness, weight loss, constipation, poor appetite, headache, and confusion, though this is unlikely to occur from eating vitamin D food sources. Toxicity is more likely to occur from taking too much of a supplement, such as cod liver oil. Appendix 3 lists your child's RDA and UL for vitamin D.

Vitamin E

Vitamin E is a fat-soluble vitamin that exists in eight different forms, with **alpha-tocopherol** the most active form. It works to support the immune system and has powerful antioxidant properties that protect cells against the damaging effects of free radicals that may contribute to chronic diseases and cancer. Its antioxidant properties also work to protect the brain and central nervous system. A vitamin E deficiency can result in peripheral neuropathy (the degeneration of nerves in the hands and feet) and increase the risk of cancer, Alzheimer's disease, and heart disease. Even the slightest vitamin E deficiency can impair your child's immune function. Here are some vitamin E–rich foods:

wheat germ   vegetable oils

nuts and seeds   green leafy vegetables

Too much vitamin E isn't toxic, but since it acts as an anticoagulant, taking an excess amount can increase the risk of prolonged bleeding. Appendix 3 lists your child's RDA and UL for vitamin E.

SUPPLEMENTS TO ENHANCE THE DETOXIFICATION SYSTEM

- Alpha-Lipoic Acid

- Glutathione

- N-acetylcysteine (NAC)

- Selenium

- Trimethylglycine (TMG)

- Vitamin C

Many people in the autism community also believe that autistic children have a dysfunctional detoxification system within their liver. The theory goes that an autistic child's liver can't effectively excrete toxins such as mercury, lead, arsenic, pesticides, herbicides, certain solvents, and other chemicals. Toxins that aren't excreted can cross the blood-brain barrier, cling to brain tissue, and damage the brain; therefore autistic children are more vulnerable to neurological damage caused by exposure to these toxins. Neurotoxin chemicals are particularly dangerous to the rapidly developing brain of a fetus, infant, and young child. Exposure to neurotoxins at these vulnerable times may result in learning disabilities, attention deficit, hyperactivity, impulsiveness, aggressive behavior, speech delay, lower I.Q., and mental retardation. To learn more about neurotoxins and the impact they can have on your child, I recommend you read the report "In Harm's Way: Toxic Threats to Child Development," which you can find at www.igc.org/psr. This excellent resource discusses the environmental factors that contribute to learning, behavioral, and developmental disabilities in our children.

Chelation Therapy

Physicians who use alternative and complementary interventions to treat autism often recommend a highly controversial treatment called chelation therapy. In chelation therapy, a drug that binds to heavy metals in the blood, such as EDTA, DMSA, or DMPS, is infused intravenously into your child's body to help eliminate toxins through urine and stool. Chelation therapy is typically used to treat mercury and lead poisoning that involves life-threatening high levels; not chronic, low-level exposure to toxins. This treatment method is controversial because little scientific research has been done to establish its effectiveness to treat autism, and it may pose serious risks to your child. Chelation therapy can lead to mineral depletion, the rupture of blood cells, liver damage, and bone marrow suppression. Some children have died because of medication errors. If you decide to try chelation therapy, your child's kidney and liver function and blood composition has to be closely monitored to avoid potential damage.

The effects of chronic, low-level exposure to multiple toxic chemicals on your child should be taken seriously, but I recommend you consider a less controversial treatment. Vitamins, minerals, sulfur-containing amino acids, nutraceuticals, and dietary modifications can all work to naturally enhance your child's detoxification system. Turn to Appendix 6 on page 237 for my comprehensive nutritional plan to enhance detoxification, which includes reducing exposure to toxins, following a protective diet, and choosing nutrients to support your child's detoxification function.

Alpha-Lipoic Acid

Alpha-lipoic acid is a disulfide compound found in plant and animal sources. It functions as an antioxidant, helps the immune system, and may have anti-aging effects. Alpha-lipoic acid plays a critical role in the detoxification system as a precursor to L-cysteine and recycler of **glutathione**, an important antioxidant that helps eliminate toxins from the body. In fact, alpha-lipoic acid actually has the ability to *increase* glutathione levels in the body. Here are some alpha–lipoic acid–rich foods:

organ meats	broccoli	Brussels sprouts
spinach	peas	tomatoes

There's been no report of adverse reactions to taking too much alpha-lipoic acid. Still, you should consult with your child's registered dietitian or physician for dosage recommendations. I suggest dosages suggested in the PDR for Nutritional Supplements.

Glutathione

Glutathione is a tripeptide made within the body from the amino acids cysteine, gluta-mate, and glycine. As I mentioned above, glutathione is critical for your child's detoxifica-tion system. It's a cofactor for the glutathione S-transferase enzymes involved in the detoxification of chemical toxins. It also functions as an antioxidant and helps the im-mune system work properly. Glutathione in supplement form is not well-absorbed in the gastrointestinal tract, so it's not usually recommended as an oral supplement. The way around this problem is to take the precursors—that is, the molecules the body needs to make glutathione—rather than glutathione itself. The major precursors of glutathione are L-cysteine and N-acetylcysteine (NAC), both of which are available in supplement form. The glutathione precursor cysteine is found in high-protein foods such as the following:

| beef | turkey | whey protein | milk |
| pork | eggs | chicken | |

There've been no reports of adverse reactions to taking too much glutathione orally. However, medical professionals advise using caution with L-cysteine supplements because no long-term safety studies have been done. In fact, most medical practitioners suggest that children avoid L-cysteine in supplement form. NAC is the preferred supplement for both adults and children because the body absorbs it better than glutathione. NAC sup-plements can cause nausea, vomiting, diarrhea, headache, and rashes. If you're interested in supplementing your child with NAC, it's crucial that you discuss dosage with his regis-tered dietitian or physician, who may refer to the PDR for Nutritional Supplements.

Trimethylglycine (TMG)

Trimethylglycine, also known as **betaine**, is a water-soluble substance related to choline. An important function of TMG is its ability to donate a methyl group and convert hom-cysteine to methionine, which is then converted to **S-Adenosyl-L-Methionine (SAMe)**. SAMe may have a positive effect on mood, emotional well-being, and depression. SAMe may also play a role in detoxification by increasing glutathione levels in the liver. (Please note: SAMe in supplement form is not recommended for use in children.) TMG works closely with other methyl donors, such as choline, folic acid, vitamin B_{12}, and SAMe, and it plays an important role in the production of carnitine. Once TMG has donated a methyl group, it becomes DMG, which has also been identified as having potential posi-tive benefits in autistic children (see page 133 for more on DMG). Trimethylglycine can be found in foods such as sugar beets, spinach, wheat, and shellfish.

There are no reports of adverse reactions to a TMG overdose, but some people have reported experiencing nausea, vomiting, and diarrhea. Experts estimate that people who eat a regular diet that contains whole wheat and seafood get approximately 100–1,000 mg of TMG per day, so if you want to conduct a trial response of supplemental TMG, I suggest basing your child's dosage amount on what's found in a typical diet. I also encourage you to discuss specific dosages for your child with his dietitian or physician.

OTHER SUPPLEMENTS OF INTEREST

- Carnosine   • Dimethylglycine (DMG)   • Flavonoid   • Vitamin B_{12}

These supplements have generated a lot of interest in the autism community, as many parents and medical practitioners have found them beneficial for autistic children. If you're interested in trying your child on one or more of these supplements, do a one-month trial response to determine if he's a positive responder or not. If you find the supplement isn't helping your child, stop giving it to him.

Carnosine

Carnosine is a dipeptide (a combination of two amino acids—alanine and histidine) that's highly concentrated in brain and muscle tissue. It functions as a powerful antioxidant, protecting the body from free radicals, and also plays a part in neurotransmission. It's sold as a supplement under the name L-carnosine. An eight-week research study in 2002 published in the *Journal of Child Neurology* reported that children with autism who were supplemented with 400 mg of L-carnosine twice a day showed improvement in behavior, socialization, communication, and an increase in their language comprehension. Carnosine can be found in meat, poultry, and fish.

Too much L-carnosine can result in irritability, hyperactivity, and insomnia. If you want to try your child on an L-carnosine supplement, you should do so only under medical supervision.

Flavonoid

Flavonoid, or bioflavonoid, refers to a class of compounds found in plants. They are known most commonly for their antioxidant properties, but recent research has shown that flavonoids also have anticancer, antimicrobial, anti-allergic, and anti-inflammatory properties. The most common flavonoid used to treat autism is **oligomeric proanthocyanidins (OPC)**. It's thought to improve the symptoms of ADHD, but there have been few research studies done to substantiate this belief. Flavonoids can be found in citrus fruits, berries, tea, ginkgo biloba, red wine, and dark chocolate.

Only a small amount of flavonoid is necessary for health benefits. Taking too much in a dietary supplement not only provides no additional benefit; it may actually be harmful. If you want to see if supplemental OPC improves your child's

ADHD symptoms, talk to his registered dietitian or physician about dosage before starting a one-month trial-response.

Vitamin B$_{12}$

Vitamin B$_{12}$ in the form of methylcobalamin, also known as methyl-B$_{12}$, has become a very popular supplemental nutritional intervention for autism. It's theorized that autistic children may have abnormalities in their methylation pathways, which affect their bodies' ability to maintain the myelin sheath (the layer of insulation covering the axon of nerve cells in the brain) and produce neurotransmitters. Vitamin B$_{12}$, folic acid, and vitamin B$_6$ (in the form of pyridoxal 5 phosphate) work in conjunction with each other to convert **homocysteine** to methionine, which is then converted to S-adenosylmethionine (SAMe). SAMe is the major methyl group donor in methylation reactions. Since vitamin B$_{12}$ is a key cofactor in methylation, large doses of the vitamin may help correct abnormalities in your child's methylation pathway.

Vitamin B$_{12}$ is difficult for the body to absorb through the gastrointestinal tract. Those who have a gastrointestinal disorder, an intrinsic factor deficiency, low hydrochloric acid in the stomach, bacterial overgrowth in the small intestines, parasites, an inflammatory bowel disorder, or gastrointestinal problems such as chronic diarrhea and inflammation have even greater trouble absorbing B$_{12}$ and are particularly at risk for a deficiency. If your child has a B$_{12}$ deficiency, he may experience symptoms such as weight loss, loss of appetite, diarrhea, constipation, abdominal pain, and a burning sensation in his tongue called **glossitis**. He may also experience cognitive changes and memory loss. Vitamin B$_{12}$ can be found in egg yolks, clams, oysters, crabs, sardines, salmon, and fortified cereals.

Unlike the other supplements I've discussed, methyl-B$_{12}$ is administered by injection to maximize absorption within the body. There have been anecdotal reports of remarkable improvements in autistic children taking methyl-B$_{12}$ injections, but so far there's been no supporting evidence from published research studies. If you want your child to try a trial response of high dosage methyl-B$_{12}$ injections, discuss it first with his physician.

Supplements Can Be Toxic

It's extremely difficult to take in too much of a vitamin or mineral through diet alone, but supplements are a different story. To avoid the risk of toxicity, do not exceed your child's UL for a particular vitamin or mineral unless his registered dietitian or physician recommends it and is monitoring his progress. Also, make sure that any potential adverse reactions are clearly explained to you.

PROJECT NO. 10

1. As you read through this chapter, make a list of the supplements that might benefit your child based on his symptoms.

2. Take your list to your child's registered dietitian or physician and discuss which supplements are appropriate for him. Here's a list of questions I suggest you ask regarding the supplements I discuss in this chapter:

   • Which of these nutrients can my child get from food?

   • Is my child already getting enough of any of these nutrients from his current multivitamin and mineral supplement?

   • Are there any lab tests required prior to taking the supplements? (Basic lab tests are listed in Appendix 7.)

   Regarding each individual supplement you're considering for your child:

   • What type of symptom relief should I expect?

   • Are there any potential side effects or adverse reactions?

   • Are there any potential interactions with my child's medications?

   • What is a safe and effective dosage for my child?

   • How long should he take the supplement?

   • How do I assess the effectiveness of the supplement?

   • Is this particular supplement intended for short-term or long-term use?

   • When should I discontinue the supplement?

3. Together, develop a plan to incorporate the supplements you choose to try into your child's current nutritional care plan.

Congratulations—you've reached the end of my 10-Step Nutrition Plan, and hopefully you've seen some exciting and encouraging improvement in your child's symptoms. Keep in mind that, as with any treatment, some of these nutritional interventions will be very helpful for your child and some will not. Improving your child's nutritional status is an ongoing and often slow process. But if you're consistent, patient, and maintain a positive attitude, you will find the right nutritional path for your child. Enjoy the journey!

PART II
GLUTEN- AND CASEIN-FREE
RECIPES FOR KID-FRIENDLY FOODS

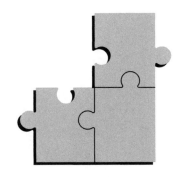

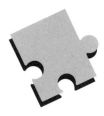

The Gluten Free Casein Free Diet is one of the most challenging nutritional interventions you'll face in my 10-Step Nutrition Plan. Gluten and casein are found in most of the prepackaged, processed foods commonly consumed by autistic children, so finding "safe" foods that will appeal to your child can be tough. To help you make your child's transition to the GFCF diet as easy and tasty as possible, this section includes more than seventy kid-friendly, gluten- and casein-free recipes that cover a wide range of main courses, beverages, breads, crackers, desserts, and condiments. Best of all, you'll find gluten- and casein-free alternatives to many of your child's favorites dishes, such as pizza, chicken nuggets, and macaroni and cheese.

As with all elimination diets, your goal is not just to eliminate foods that contain "unsafe" ingredients, but to replace these food with healthier alternatives To this end, these recipes were designed to provide your child with healthy alternatives, free not only of gluten and casein, but also of soy, refined white sugar, trans-fatty acids, and artificial chemicals. Additionally, many of the recipes include ingredients that will naturally increase your child's intake of healthy omega-3 fatty acids. (An added bonus: Since it can be very difficult to get autistic children to eat their veggies, page 210 has a recipe for a vegetable puree that you can "sneak" into many different recipes to increase your child's nutrient intake.)

Delicious, nutritious, and easy to make, these recipes will help make the GFCF diet an adventure your child—and your entire family—can enjoy!

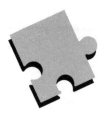

Beverages

HOT CHOCOLATE

Serves 1

This recipe was tested using West Soy Organic Unsweetened Soymilk and Nature's Place Organic Original Rice milk. If using a brand that contains a sweetener, you will need to reduce the amount of stevia used. Please note that the version prepared with rice milk was preferred.

   1 cup unsweetened soymilk or rice milk
   or ⅓ cup coconut milk combined with ⅔ cup water
   ⅛ teaspoon stevia
   1½ teaspoons cocoa
   ⅛ teaspoon vanilla
   1 tablespoon coconut milk
      (optional, but adds a little creaminess)

Combine all ingredients in a microwave-safe mug. Stir well. Microwave on high for approximately 1½ minutes.

CREAMY ORANGE SHAKE

Makes approximately 3½ cups

This recipe is fashioned after the famous Orange Julius beverage. It is an almost-frozen, frothy orange drink. Try the strawberry version, too!

    2 cups ice cubes
    1½ cups orange juice (fortified with calcium)
    2 tablespoons powdered egg whites (Deb El Just Whites)
    1 teaspoon vanilla
    ¼ teaspoon xanthan gum

Combine all ingredients in a blender. Puree until smooth. Serve right away.

CREAMY STRAWBERRY SHAKE

Makes approximately 4½ cups

This recipe has great strawberry flavor, and it was preferred over orange by our taste-testers.

    2 cups ice cubes
    2 cups fresh strawberries
    2 tablespoons honey
    1 cup very cold water (filtered)
    2 tablespoons powdered egg whites (Deb El Just Whites)
    1 teaspoon lemon juice
    ¼ teaspoon xanthan gum

Combine all ingredients in blender. Puree until smooth. Serve right away.

LEMONADE

Serves 1

juice from 1 lemon or ¼ cup lemon juice
1 cup cold water (filtered)
½ teaspoon stevia or 1 tablespoon honey

Combine all ingredients in a tall glass. Fill glass with ice.

SMOOTHIE (WITH DAIRY-FREE YOGURT)

Makes 3½ cups

Using frozen fruit makes this a milkshake-like treat. The vanilla flavoring adds a subtle undertone that enhances the flavor.

1 cup plain, coconut, or other dairy-free yogurt
¼ teaspoon vanilla
2 cups fresh or frozen fruit
1 cup orange juice (fortified with calcium)
2 tablespoons honey

Combine all ingredients in a blender. Puree until smooth.

SMOOTHIE

Makes approximately 3 cups

Coconut milk adds a creaminess to this smoothie.

½ cup coconut milk (or other dairy-free milk)
½ teaspoon vanilla
2 cups fresh or frozen fruit
1 cup orange juice (fortified with calcium)
2 tablespoons honey

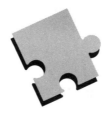

Breads and Muffins

BISCUITS

Makes 6 to 8

These biscuits are tender and not too sweet with a mild, whole grain flavor. Using coconut or other dairy-free yogurt instead of apple juice softens the flavor.

½ cup brown rice flour, 65 grams
½ cup sorghum flour, 65 grams
1 tablespoon flax seed meal (optional)
2 teaspoons Rumford baking powder
1 teaspoon baking soda
½ teaspoon salt

1½ teaspoons xanthan gum
½ cup trans fat-free shortening
½ cup plain, coconut, or other dairy-free yogurt or ½ cup apple juice
2 tablespoons honey
1 tablespoon apple cider vinegar

Preheat oven to 375 °F. Lightly grease a baking sheet.

In a medium-size bowl, combine all dry ingredients. Stir. Add shortening and mix until mixture resembles a fine crumb. Add juice, honey, and vinegar. Mix well until combined into a pasty, soft dough. It will be quite fragile.

Pat out dough on the baking sheet to ½-inch thickness. Cut into square biscuits and push apart with the side of the knife.

Bake for 15 to 20 minutes, depending upon thickness, until the biscuits have browned and are cooked through.

BREAD LOAF

Makes 12 small slices

This bread is light in flavor with a tight crumb. Although not tall in height, you will enjoy its springy texture.

⅔ cup brown rice flour, 80 grams
⅓ cup sorghum flour, 45 grams
⅓ cup canola oil
1 tablespoon flaxseed meal
2 tablespoons honey
1 teaspoon apple cider vinegar
2 eggs (omega-3 enriched)
1 tablespoon Rumford baking powder
½ teaspoon baking soda
1 teaspoon xanthan gum
½ teaspoon salt
½ cup apple juice

Preheat oven to 350 °F. Lightly grease a medium-size loaf pan.

In a mixing bowl, combine flours and oil. Mix well to combine. Add remaining ingredients and mix well. Batter will thicken as it is beaten. Pour into loaf pan. Smooth top with moistened fingertips for prettier loaf, if desired.

Bake for approximately 30 minutes, until a toothpick inserted in the middle tests clean.

EASY DINNER ROLLS

Makes 12

These rolls are baked in a muffin tin for quick and easy preparation. They are light and savory.

⅔ cup brown rice flour, 80 grams
⅓ cup sorghum flour, 45 grams
⅓ cup canola oil
2 tablespoons honey
1 teaspoon apple cider vinegar
2 eggs (omega-3 enriched)
1 tablespoon Rumford baking powder
½ teaspoon baking soda
¾ teaspoon xanthan gum
½ teaspoon cinnamon
½ teaspoon salt
½ cup apple juice

Topping (optional):
1 teaspoon ground flaxseed meal

Preheat oven to 350 °F. Lightly grease a muffin tin.

In a mixing bowl, combine flours and oil. Mix well to combine. Add the remaining ingredients and mix well. Batter will thicken as it is beaten.

Divide batter among twelve cups in the tin. Bake for approximately 15 to 18 minutes, until a toothpick inserted in the middle tests clean.

FLATBREAD

Makes 4

This flatbread is soft and quite flat. They are ideal for sandwiches and fajitas.

> 2 egg whites
> 1 tablespoon canola oil
> ½ cup apple juice
> ¼ cup brown rice flour, 35 grams
> ¼ cup sorghum flour, 35 grams
> ¼ teaspoon baking soda
> ¼ teaspoon salt
> 1 ¾ teaspoons xanthan gum

Preheat oven to 350 °F. Lightly grease a baking sheet.

Place the egg whites in a medium-size bowl. Beat until very frothy. Add the remaining ingredients. Mix well. The dough will look very soft and stretchy.

Drop dough by ¼ cup onto the baking sheet. Using wet fingertips, spread the dough as thin as possible, approximately ⅛-inch thickness—a 10-inch circle is a good size. Bake for 10 to 12 minutes, until the bottom of the dough is lightly browned and the edges of the flatbread begin to color lightly.

HOT DOG ROLLS AND HAMBURGER BUNS

Serves 4

This recipe makes four nicely sized rolls or buns. While whole grain, they are mild in flavor.

> **3 egg whites**
> **1 tablespoon canola oil**
> **½ cup unsweetened applesauce**
> **¼ cup apple juice**
> **½ cup brown rice flour, 65 grams**
> **½ cup sorghum flour, 65 grams**
> **2 teaspoons Rumford baking powder**
> **1 teaspoon baking soda**
> **½ teaspoon salt**
> **1 teaspoon xanthan gum**
> **1 tablespoon apple cider vinegar**

Preheat oven to 350 °F. Lightly grease a baking sheet.

In a medium-size bowl, beat the egg whites until very frothy. Add the remaining ingredients. Mix well. Batter will be light and pillowy. Place the dough into a large, square plastic bag. Snip one corner off the bottom edge of the bag, approximately 1½ inches wide.

Pipe hot dog rolls or hamburger buns onto the prepared pan. Bake approximately 20 minutes until the rolls are lightly browned and test cleanly with a toothpick. Cool. Slice in half (nearly through) before serving.

PIZZA CRUST

Makes one large or four individual crusts

You can actually see the soft, breadlike texture of this crust as you pat out the dough. When it's spread to 10 inches, it yields a hand-tossed crust. Spread thicker or thinner according to your own taste.

3 egg whites
1 tablespoon olive oil
½ cup apple juice
¼ cup brown rice flour, 35 grams
¼ cup sorghum flour, 35 grams
2 teaspoons Rumford baking powder
¼ teaspoon baking soda
¼ teaspoon salt
1 ¾ teaspoons xanthan gum

Preheat oven to 350 °F. Lightly grease a baking sheet.

Place the egg whites in a medium-size bowl. Beat until very frothy. Add the remaining ingredients. Mix well. The dough will look like very soft cookie dough.

Drop dough onto prepared pan. Using wet fingertips, spread the dough to ¼-inch thickness—a 10-inch circle is a good size. Bake for 10 to 15 minutes, until the bottom of the dough is lightly browned and the edges of the crust begin to color lightly. (Bake longer for a crisper crust.)

Raise the oven temperature to 400 °F.

Top the partially baked crust with ⅔ cup of pizza sauce (page 186) and 1 cup of shredded dairy-free cheese (or other desired toppings). Bake until the crust is golden and cheese is melted (and just beginning to brown), 5 to 10 minutes.

TORTILLAS, RICE

Makes 6

Adapted from the recipe for traditional corn tortillas in the *Joy of Cooking*, these tortillas use brown rice flour (the coarser the better). Use these tortillas in tacos or for making tortilla chips or in your favorite Mexican dish. Do not be concerned if your tortillas are not quite perfect circles. The flavor of these tortillas is very mild and requires little or no browning.

1½ cups brown rice flour, 190 grams
½ cup hot water (filtered)
¼ teaspoon salt

Mix together to form a dough. If crumbly, add a little more hot water. Cover dough with plastic. Allow dough to rest for 30 minutes.

Divide dough into 6 pieces. Roll in a circle shape as thin as possible, no more than ¹⁄₁₆ inch thick. For rolling, place the dough between two pieces of heavy plastic, such as the cut-away sides of a zip-type bag. If dough sticks to the plastic, add a little more brown rice flour. The dough should feel like very dry, gritty Play-Doh.

Note: Should you be using these to make tortilla chips, it is very important that the dough be rolled as thin as possible.

Heat a large frying pan or griddle over high heat. Add one tortilla at a time, cooking for approximately 30 seconds on each side. The underside of the tortilla will blister slightly, forming air pockets.

APPLESAUCE MUFFINS

Makes 12

Light and moist. For blueberry muffins, omit the cinnamon and fold in 1 cup of fresh or frozen berries after mixing.

½ cup brown rice flour, 65 grams
½ cup sorghum flour, 65 grams
⅓ cup canola oil
½ cup unsweetened applesauce
½ cup honey
1 teaspoon apple cider vinegar
½ teaspoon vanilla
2 eggs (omega-3 enriched)
1 tablespoon Rumford baking powder
½ teaspoon baking soda
½ teaspoon xanthan gum
½ teaspoon cinnamon
½ teaspoon salt

Preheat oven to 350 °F. Place muffin liners in a muffin tin.

In a mixing bowl, combine flours and oil. Mix well to combine. Add remaining ingredients and mix well. Batter will thicken as it is beaten.

Divide batter among twelve liners. Bake for approximately 15 to 18 minutes, until a toothpick inserted in the middle tests clean.

BANANA MUFFINS

Makes 12

These muffins have a wonderful, mild flavor. Not too sweet, soft, and moist. The foil muffin liners are especially nice for lining your pan.

   2 small bananas mashed, ¾ cup
   ½ cup brown rice flour, 65 grams
   ½ cup sorghum flour, 65 grams
   ⅓ cup canola oil
   ½ cup honey
   1 teaspoon apple cider vinegar
   1 teaspoon vanilla
   2 eggs (omega-3 enriched)
   1 tablespoon Rumford baking powder
   ½ teaspoon baking soda
   ¾ teaspoon xanthan gum
   ½ teaspoon salt

Preheat oven to 350 °F. Place muffin liners in muffin tins.

Mash bananas in a small bowl. Set aside.

In a mixing bowl, combine flours and oil. Mix well. Add the remaining ingredients, including bananas, and mix well. Batter will thicken a little as it is beaten.

Divide batter among 12 liners. Bake for approximately 18 to 20 minutes, until a toothpick inserted in the middle tests clean.

DOUBLE CHOCOLATE MUFFINS

Makes 12

My kids love double chocolate muffins. These mix up quickly and are sure to be a favorite snack. It is difficult to eat just one.

½ cup brown rice flour, 65 grams
¼ cup sorghum flour, 35 grams
⅓ cup canola oil
⅓ cup cocoa, 30 grams
½ cup unsweetened applesauce
½ cup honey
1 teaspoon vanilla
2 eggs (omega-3 enriched)
1 teaspoon Rumford baking powder
1 teaspoon baking soda
½ teaspoon xanthan gum
½ teaspoon salt
1 cup GFCF semisweet chocolate chips

Preheat oven to 350 °F. Place muffin liners in muffin tins.

In a mixing bowl, combine brown rice flour, sorghum flour, and oil. Mix well. Add the remaining ingredients, except the chips, and mix well. Batter will thicken as it is beaten. Fold in the chips.

Divide batter among 12 liners. Bake for approximately 17 to 21 minutes, until a toothpick inserted in the middle tests clean.

PUMPKIN MUFFINS

Makes 12

Light, moist and mildly spiced, these muffins are good for breakfast or just a snack. The cinnamon may be omitted if it is not a favorite flavor.

½ cup brown rice flour, 65 grams
½ cup sorghum flour, 65 grams
⅓ cup canola oil
½ cup pumpkin (canned)
½ cup honey
1 teaspoon apple cider vinegar
½ teaspoon vanilla
2 eggs (omega-3 enriched)
1 tablespoon Rumford baking powder
½ teaspoon baking soda
½ teaspoon xanthan gum
½ teaspoon cinnamon
½ teaspoon salt

Preheat oven to 350 °F. Place muffin liners in muffin tins.

In a mixing bowl, combine flours and oil. Mix well. Add the remaining ingredients and mix well. Batter will thicken as it is beaten.

Divide batter among 12 liners. Bake for approximately 15 to 18 minutes, until a toothpick inserted in the middle tests clean.

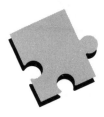

Breakfasts

FRENCH TOAST

Makes 6 slices

Rice milk provides a nice base for this dish. A little vanilla and cinnamon make it a traditional favorite.

  2 eggs (omega-3 enriched)
  ½ cup rice milk
  1 tablespoon honey
  2 teaspoons canola oil
  ¼ teaspoon vanilla
  ¼ teaspoon cinnamon
  pinch of xanthan gum
  6 slices gluten-free bread

In a medium-size bowl, combine all ingredients, except bread, and mix well. Over medium heat, heat the frying pan. Lightly grease pan if it's not nonstick.

Dip slices of bread into the batter and place in the pan. Cook on each side for a minute or two to brown. The exterior should be slightly crisp but not burnt. Turn and cook on other side. Serve hot.

GRANOLA

Makes approximately 4½ cups

This simple granola is a little sweet with a touch of vanilla flavor.

¼ cup canola oil
½ cup honey
½ teaspoon vanilla
2 cups gluten-free rolled oats
1 tablespoon flax seed meal
½ cup sliced almonds
1 small apple, cored, peeled, and finely diced
½ cup raisins

Preheat oven to 350 °F. Lightly grease baking sheet.

In a large bowl combine oil, honey, and vanilla. Mix well. Add the remaining ingredients, except raisins. Mix until well coated. Pour onto the prepared pan and bake for 40 to 50 minutes, until lightly browned. Turn the granola once or twice during baking. Remove from the oven and stir in raisins. Allow to cool fully on the baking sheet.

PANCAKES

Makes eight 4-inch pancakes

These pancakes taste like a light, whole grain pancake. Be sure to allow pancakes to rest for a minute or so after cooking. Otherwise, the pancakes seem too moist.

½ cup brown rice flour, 65 grams
½ cup sorghum flour, 65 grams
1 tablespoon flax seed meal
1 tablespoon baking powder
½ teaspoon xanthan gum
½ teaspoon salt
2 eggs (omega-3 enriched)
¼ cup canola oil
1 tablespoon honey
½ teaspoon vanilla extract
¾ cup apple juice

Heat a pan or griddle to low-medium heat.

Place all dry ingredients in a medium-size bowl. Stir well to combine. Add the remaining ingredients and mix well. The batter will become quite thick as it sits. Pour the batter in the pan or griddle to your desired size of pancakes. Spread with the back of a spoon if necessary.

Cook until small bubbles appear on the surface and the bottom is lightly browned. Flip and continue to cook until lightly browned on both sides.

Allow pancakes to rest for a minute prior to serving.

WAFFLES

Makes six 8-inch waffles

These waffles are medium-textured with an almost-nutty undertone. Just one waffle is quite satisfying. Reheat extras in the toaster.

¾ cup brown rice flour, 95 grams
¾ cup sorghum flour, 100 grams
1 tablespoon flax seed meal
1 tablespoon plus 1 teaspoon baking powder
½ teaspoon xanthan gum
½ teaspoon salt
3 eggs (omega-3 enriched)
⅓ cup canola oil
2 tablespoons honey
1 teaspoon vanilla extract
¾ cup apple juice

Heat waffle iron.

Place all dry ingredients in a medium-size bowl. Stir well to combine. Add the remaining ingredients and mix well. The batter will be very thick. Pour a large ½ cup of batter onto a waffle iron. Cook to desired level of browning, approximately 1½ to 2 minutes.

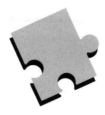

Cakes, Cookies, and Desserts

CARROT CAKE

Serves 8

We're sneaking both carrots and zucchini into this cake! It is a nice snacking cake that needs no icing. Add a handful of chopped raisins if you like.

1 cup brown rice flour, 125 grams
⅓ cup canola oil
½ teaspoon salt
½ teaspoon baking soda
2 teaspoons Rumford baking powder
½ teaspoon xanthan gum
½ cup grated carrot
½ cup grated zucchini
½ cup honey
2 eggs (omega-3 enriched)
1 teaspoon vanilla extract
½ teaspoon cinnamon (optional)

Preheat the oven to 350 °F. Lightly grease a 9-inch round or square pan.

In a medium-size bowl, combine rice flour and oil. Stir briefly. Add remaining ingredients and stir well. Batter will thicken with mixing. Spread in the prepared pan. Bake for 30 to 35 minutes, until a toothpick inserted in the middle tests clean.

CHOCOLATE CAKE

Serves 8

This cake is moist, tender, and squishy. It is delicious. Be sure to bake in a 9-inch pan with sides that are at least 2 inches tall. The cake rises near the top of the pan, then settles a little after baking. Wilton pans (available at craft stores) or commercial pans are ideal.

⅓ cup brown rice flour, 40 grams
⅓ cup sorghum flour, 45 grams
½ cup unsweetened cocoa powder, 40 grams
1 teaspoon salt
½ teaspoon baking soda
1 teaspoon Rumford baking powder
scant ½ teaspoon xanthan gum
½ cup canola oil
¾ cup plus 2 tablespoons honey
2 eggs (omega-3 enriched)
1 teaspoon vanilla extract
¼ cup water (filtered)

Preheat the oven to 350 °F. Lightly grease a 9-inch round or square pan.

In a medium-size bowl, combine all dry ingredients. Stir briefly. Add remaining ingredients and stir well. Batter will be the consistency of molasses. Spread in the prepared pan. Bake for 35 minutes, until a toothpick inserted in the middle tests clean and the top begins to appear dry.

ICING

Makes approximately ⅔ cup, enough to lightly frost one 9-inch cake

This thin icing is very sweet and should be used in smaller quantity than traditional icing. It has a definite honey taste with subtle vanilla undertones.

> ¼ cup trans fat-free shortening
> ½ cup honey
> 1 teaspoon vanilla
> ¼ teaspoon xanthan gum

In a mixing bowl, combine shortening and honey. Beat until creamy. Add the vanilla and beat well. If mixture is thin (very likely), sprinkle the top of the icing with xanthan gum. Beat until the icing thickens.

SWEET MERINGUE ICING

Makes approximately 1½ cups, enough to generously frost one 9-inch cake

This icing is like a cross between meringue and traditional icing. By using xanthan gum, we are able to stabilize the foam. And by using dried or pasteurized egg whites, we are able to avoid cooking the frosting. It is very tasty without a strong (if any) honey taste.

> 1 egg white (pasteurized or reconstituted dry egg white)
> 2 tablespoons honey
> 1 teaspoon vanilla
> ⅛ teaspoon xanthan gum

In a mixing bowl, combine egg white and honey. Beat until very frothy. Add vanilla and beat until soft peaks just begin to form. Sprinkle xanthan gum over the top and continue beating until soft and creamy. Spread over the cake.

CHOCOLATE SWEET MERINGUE ICING

Makes approximately 1½ cups, enough to generously frost one 9-inch cake

This icing is my favorite among those made without sugar. It makes a creamy, stabilized foam that adds a little extra oomph to a cake, without it being too much.

1 egg white (pasteurized or reconstituted dry egg white)
2 tablespoons honey
2 teaspoons vanilla
2 teaspoons cocoa
⅛ teaspoon xanthan gum

In a mixing bowl, combine egg white and honey. Beat until very frothy. Add vanilla and beat until soft peaks just begin to form. Beat in the cocoa. Sprinkle xanthan gum over the top and continue beating until soft and creamy. Spread over the cake.

POUND CAKE

Serves 9

This cake is moist with a mellow honey/vanilla flavor. Be sure to serve the cake nicely cooled, as hot from the oven it will be too moist. Serve this cake with fresh fruit for a special treat.

¾ cup brown rice flour, 95 grams
¼ cup sorghum flour, 35 grams
⅓ cup canola oil
½ teaspoon salt
½ teaspoon baking soda
1 teaspoon Rumford baking powder
½ teaspoon xanthan gum
¼ cup unsweetened applesauce
½ cup honey
1 tablespoon apple cider vinegar
3 eggs (omega-3 enriched)
1½ teaspoons vanilla extract

Preheat the oven to 350 °F. Lightly grease a medium-size loaf pan.

In a medium-size bowl, combine flours and oil. Stir briefly. Add the remaining ingredients and stir well. Batter will thicken with mixing. Spread in the prepared pan. Bake for approximately 45 minutes, until a toothpick inserted in the middle tests clean.

POUND CAKE, CHOCOLATE

Serves 9

This cake is very pretty. It is chocolatey and not too sweet.

½ cup brown rice flour, 65 grams
¼ cup sorghum flour, 35 grams
⅓ cup canola oil
⅓ cup cocoa, 30 grams
½ teaspoon salt
½ teaspoon baking soda
1 teaspoon Rumford baking powder
½ teaspoon xanthan gum
¼ cup unsweetened applesauce
½ cup honey
3 eggs (omega-3 enriched)
1 teaspoon vanilla extract

Preheat the oven to 350 °F. Lightly grease a medium-size loaf pan.

In a medium-size bowl, combine flours and oil. Stir briefly. Add the remaining ingredients and stir well. Batter will thicken with mixing. Spread in the prepared pan. Bake for approximately 45 minutes, until a toothpick inserted in the middle tests clean.

YELLOW CAKE

Serves 8

This cake is soft and moist. Although there is applesauce in the recipe, it tastes like a typical yellow cake.

> 1 cup brown rice flour, 125 grams
> ⅓ cup canola oil
> ½ teaspoon salt
> ½ teaspoon baking soda
> 2 teaspoons Rumford baking powder
> ½ teaspoon xanthan gum
> ½ cup unsweetened applesauce
> ½ cup honey
> 2 eggs (omega-3 enriched)
> 1 teaspoon vanilla extract

Preheat the oven to 350 °F. Lightly grease a nine-inch round or square pan.

In a medium-size bowl, combine rice flour and oil. Stir briefly. Add the remaining ingredients and stir well. Batter will thicken with mixing. Spread in the prepared pan. Bake for 30 to 35 minutes, until a toothpick inserted in the middle tests clean.

BROWNIES

Serves 8

These brownies have a tight, moist crumb. They are better at room temperature.

¼ cup brown rice flour, 30 grams
1 tablespoon flax seed meal
⅓ cup unsweetened cocoa powder, 30 grams
½ teaspoon salt
¼ teaspoon xanthan gum
¼ cup canola oil
½ cup honey
2 eggs (omega-3 enriched)
1 teaspoon vanilla extract
2 tablespoons water

Preheat the oven to 350 °F. Lightly grease a 9-inch round or square pan.

In a medium-size bowl, combine all dry ingredients. Stir briefly. Add the remaining ingredients and stir well. Batter will be the consistency of molasses. Spread in the prepared pan. Bake for 20 to 25 minutes, until a toothpick inserted in the middle tests cleanly and the top begins to appear dry.

CHOCOLATE CHIP COOKIES

Makes 36

These cookies are very tasty! The shape of the cookie changes very little during baking, making it very important not to overbeat the batter—which makes the dough stiffer. Molasses is used to add that "brown sugar" flavor in traditional chocolate chip cookies.

⅓ cup canola oil
½ cup honey
1 tablespoon unsulphured molasses
1 egg (omega-3 enriched)
¾ cup brown rice flour, 95 grams
¾ cup sorghum flour, 100 grams
½ teaspoon baking soda
2 teaspoons Rumford baking powder
½ teaspoon salt
1½ teaspoons vanilla extract
¼ cup apple juice
2¼ teaspoons xanthan gum
1 cup semi-sweet, dairy-free chocolate chips

Preheat the oven to 375 °F. Lightly grease a cookie sheet.

In a medium-size mixing bowl, combine oil, honey, molasses, and egg. Mix well until well blended. Add the remaining ingredients, except the chocolate chips. Beat until the batter blends together. Fold in the chips. Try not to overbeat, otherwise the shape of the cookies will not be pretty.

Drop dough by rounded teaspoonfuls onto a prepared pan. The shape of the cookie may be finetuned using moistened fingertips. Cookies should be no more than ¼-inch thick.

Bake for approximately 10 minutes, until lightly browned on top. Transfer from the cookie sheet to a rack and let cool completely.

CHOCOLATE COOKIES

Makes 36

These cookies have a cakelike texture and are not overly sweet. If you have a sweet tooth, fold in one cup of chocolate chips after mixing.

⅓ cup canola oil
½ cup honey
1 egg (omega-3 enriched)
¾ cup brown rice flour, 95 grams
½ cup sorghum flour, 65 grams
¼ cup cocoa, 20 grams
½ teaspoon baking soda
1 teaspoon Rumford baking powder
½ teaspoon salt
1 teaspoon vanilla extract
¼ cup apple juice
2 teaspoons xanthan gum

Preheat the oven to 375 °F. Lightly grease a cookie sheet.

In a medium-size mixing bowl, combine oil, honey, and egg. Mix until well blended. Add remaining ingredients except the chocolate chips. Beat until the batter just blends together. It will look like a thicker cake batter. Try not to overbeat; otherwise the shape of the cookies will not be pretty.

Drop dough by rounded teaspoonfuls onto prepared pan. The shape of the cookie may be fine-tuned using moistened fingertips. Cookies should be no more than ¼-inch thick.

Bake for approximately 10 minutes until cooked through. The cookie will have lost its sheen when done. Transfer from the cookie sheet to a rack and let cool completely.

CHOCOLATE FUDGE NO BAKE COOKIES

Makes 12

Be sure to use safe oats when you make these cookies! They are very rich and filling. I prefer to use thinner-cut oatmeal when available.

¼ cup canola oil
½ cup peanut butter (organic)
½ cup honey
2 tablespoons cocoa
1½ teaspoons vanilla
2 cups gluten-free oats

Lightly grease a baking sheet. Set aside.

In a medium saucepan, combine oil, peanut butter, honey, cocoa, and vanilla. Cook, stirring often, over medium heat until peanut butter melts and ingredients blend well. Mixture should boil for a minute or so. Add the oats and stir well. Drop by a rounded tablespoon onto the prepared pan.

GINGERBREAD MEN

Makes approximately 12 cookies, depending upon size

These cookies take a little time to prepare but are worth it. They may be decorated with bits of candy or icing after baking, if desired.

⅓ cup trans fat-free shortening
½ cup honey
1 tablespoon unsulphured molasses
¾ cup brown rice flour, 95 grams
¾ cup sorghum flour, 100 grams
½ teaspoon baking soda
½ teapoon baking powder
1 teaspoon ginger
¼ teaspoon cinnamon
½ teaspoon salt
1 teaspoon xanthan gum

Preheat the oven to 375 °F. Lightly grease a cookie sheet.

In a medium-size bowl, combine shortening, honey and molasses. Beat well to combine. Add remaining ingredients and beat well. Batter will be thick and pasty.

Place one rounded tablespoon of dough onto prepared pan. Spread to ⅛ inch (or less) thickness. (Moistened fingertips make this task easier.) Use a cookie cutter to cut the shape of the cookies. Remove excess dough and recycle for additional cookies.

Bake for approximately 13 minutes, until top is nicely browned. If taken out too soon, the cookies will remain bendable instead of crisping.

PEANUT BUTTER COOKIES

Makes 36 cookies

These peanut butter cookies are not too sweet and are mild in flavor. Add a little extra honey or 1 teaspoon of stevia if you prefer a sweeter-tasting cookie.

- ¼ cup canola oil
- ½ cup peanut butter (organic)
- ½ cup honey
- 1 egg (omega-3 enriched)
- 1 teaspoon apple cider vinegar
- ¾ cup brown rice flour, 95 grams
- ½ cup sorghum flour, 65 grams
- ½ teaspoon baking soda
- 1 tablespoon Rumford baking powder
- ½ teaspoon salt
- 1½ teaspoons vanilla extract
- 2¼ teaspoons xanthan gum

Preheat the oven to 375 °F. Lightly grease a cookie sheet.

In a medium-size mixing bowl, combine oil, peanut butter, honey, and egg. Mix well, until light and thick. Add the remaining ingredients. Beat until a shiny-looking dough forms. Try not to overbeat (beyond when dough forms), otherwise the shape of the cookies will not be as pretty.

Shape teaspoonfuls of dough into 1-inch balls. Place onto the prepared pan. Press with tines of fork twice to form a crisscross pattern on top of cookie. (If fork sticks, you may dip the fork into brown rice flour before each press onto the dough.) Cookie should be no more than ¼-inch thick.

Bake for approximately 10 minutes, until lightly browned at the bottom edges. Transfer from the cookie sheet to a rack and let cool completely.

SUGAR COOKIES

Makes 36

These sugar cookies may be sprinkled with a bit of unrefined sugar to mimic traditional "sprinkles." These cookies are soft and mild in flavor.

⅓ cup trans fat-free shortening
½ cup honey
1 ¼ cups brown rice flour, 125 grams
¼ cup sorghum flour, 35 grams
½ teaspoon baking soda
1 egg (omega-3 enriched)
½ teaspoon salt
1 teaspoon vanilla
1 teaspoon xanthan gum

Topping (optional):
unrefined sugar

Preheat the oven to 375 °F. Lightly grease a cookie sheet.

In medium-size bowl, combine shortening and honey. Beat well to combine. Add remaining ingredients and beat well. Batter will be soft and pasty.

Place one rounded tablespoon of dough at a time onto prepared pan. Press with the bottom of a glass that's been dipped in water to flatten to ¼ inch, or leave alone for a domed top. (Either way is very good.) Sprinkle tops lightly with unrefined sugar, if desired.

Bake for approximately 8 to 10 minutes, until tops are nicely browned.

Move cookies to cooling rack to cool completely. Cookies will crisp as they cool.

PUDDING, CHOCOLATE

Serves 4

Soft, creamy, and pleasant.

    2 cups plain rice milk
    2 teaspoons xanthan gum
    2 tablespoons cocoa
    1 teaspoon vanilla
    scant ½ teaspoon stevia
    1 teaspoon canola oil
    1 egg (omega-3 enriched)

Place all ingredients in a medium-size saucepan. Bring this to a near boil over medium heat. Stir often. Mixture will thicken more upon cooling.

FRUIT GELATIN

Serves 4

Very flavorful fruit is the secret to good results with this recipe. Frozen mixed berries are a nice choice. Very ripe strawberries make a subtle, pleasant flavor. Additional sweetener may be needed if the fruit is not very ripe.

    1 cup water (filtered)
    1 envelope unflavored gelatin
    1 cup fresh fruit or frozen mixed berries
    ½ cup water (filtered) or 100 percent juice
    2 tablespoons honey or ¼ teaspoon stevia powder

Place water in a small saucepan or microwave-safe bowl. Sprinkle gelatin over the water. Allow to stand for one minute. Heat (or microwave) and stir until water boils and gelatin is dissolved.

   Place fruit, liquid, and sweetener in a blender. Puree until smooth. Add to gelatin mixture. Refrigerate until set.

ICE CREAM, BERRY

Makes 3 cups in a home freezer

Although not truly an ice cream, this frozen treat is wonderful. Because frozen fruit is used, the freezing time is cut considerably.

>   8 ounces frozen mixed berries
>   1½ cups rice milk
>   1 tablespoon canola oil
>   ¼ cup honey
>   ½ teaspoon xanthan gum

Place all ingredients in a blender and blend well. Pour into a freezer-safe bowl and freeze for approximately one hour. Stir well and return to the freezer. Continue stirring each hour until the ice cream is the desired texture. Store covered until serving.

Once blended, the mixture may also be placed into an ice cream freezer. This will make a lighter, airier ice cream.

ICE CREAM, CHOCOLATE

Makes 3 cups in a home freezer

Very rich and chocolately, and is a cross between a sorbet and an ice cream.

>   2 ¼ cups rice milk
>   1 tablespoon canola oil
>   2 tablespoons cocoa
>   ¼ cup honey
>   1 teaspoon vanilla
>   ½ teaspoon xanthan gum

Place all ingredients in a blender and blend well. Pour into a freezer-safe bowl and freeze for approximately one hour. Stir well and return to the freezer. Continue stirring each hour until the ice cream is the desired texture. Store covered until serving.

Once blended, the mixture may also be placed into an ice cream freezer. This will make it a lighter, airier ice cream.

ICE CREAM, PEACH

Makes 3 cups in home freezer

Frozen peaches bring you season-fresh taste in this ice cream.

    8 ounces frozen peaches
    1½ cups rice milk
    1 tablespoon canola oil
    ¼ cup honey
    1 teaspoon vanilla
    ½ teaspoon xanthan gum

Place all ingredients in a blender and blend well. Pour into a freezer-safe bowl and freeze for approximately one hour. Stir well and return to the freezer. Continue stirring each hour until the ice cream is the desired texture. Store covered until serving.

    Once blended, the mixture may also be placed into an ice cream freezer. This will make for lighter, airier ice cream.

PUDDING, VANILLA

Serves 4

This soft, creamy pudding is reminiscent of tapioca without the little lumps. The rice milk provides a mild undertone while the egg (technically making this a custard) adds body to the pudding.

    2 cups plain rice milk
    2 teaspoons xanthan gum
    1 teaspoon vanilla
    scant ½ teaspoon stevia
    1 teaspoon canola oil
    1 egg (omega-3 enriched)

Place all ingredients in a medium-size saucepan. Over medium heat, bring to a near boil. Stir often. The mixture will thicken more upon cooling.

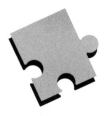

Condiments and Sauces

BUTTER SUBSTITUTE

Makes approximately ½ cup

For use in baking or for spreading, this substitute is very mild in flavor.

¼ cup trans fat-free shortening
3 tablespoons unsweetened applesauce
½ teaspoon lemon juice
pinch of salt

Combine all ingredients in a small cup or bowl. Mix vigorously to combine.

CATSUP

Makes approximately 3 cups

In this recipe, I recommend using Contadina brand tomato paste, as its ingredient list is very short: tomatoes. Honey is my preferred sweetener, but stevia powder is a pleasant alternative. This catsup is not quite as sweet as commercial catsups. Increase the honey by half if you desire something sweeter.

2 cups water (filtered)
two 6-ounce cans tomato paste
1 tablespoon apple cider vinegar
½ teaspoon garlic salt
½ teaspoon sea salt
¼ teaspoon paprika
1 tablespoon finely chopped onion
6 tablespoons honey *or*
   1½ teaspoons stevia powder

Combine all ingredients in a blender. Puree until smooth. Place in a medium saucepan. Bring to a boil over medium heat, stirring often. Turn down heat to a slow boil and cook for approximately 5 minutes. Refrigerate.

MAYONNAISE

Makes 1½ cups

This mayonnaise is mild in flavor. Although very nice as is, I add a little tarragon or paprika for an extra flavor boost.

1 tablespoon dried egg whites (Deb El Just Whites)
1 tablespoon apple cider vinegar
½ teaspoon salt
5 tablespoons water
1 cup canola oil

Place dried egg whites, vinegar, salt, and water in a blender. Blend until well combined. With blender running, slowly pour in oil. Scrape down the sides of the blender if needed during mixing.

RANCH-STYLE DRESSING

Makes approximately 1 ½ cups

Dairy-based ranch dressing has nothing on this version. Enjoy it on salads or for dipping.

¼ cup canola oil
½ cup mayonnaise
¼ cup coconut milk
3 tablespoons apple cider vinegar
½ teaspoon garlic salt
2 teaspoons honey or pinch of
    stevia powder

1 tablespoon minced onion
1 teaspoon lemon juice
1 teaspoon tarragon (dried)
¼ teaspoon xanthan gum

Combine all ingredients in a medium-size bowl. Stir well to combine. Mixture will thicken in a minute or two.

TACO SEASONING

Mix up a few batches of this recipe to save time.

1 tablespoon brown rice flour
1 tablespoons sorghum flour
1½ teaspoons garlic salt
1½ teaspoon chili powder
½ teaspoon onion powder
¼ teaspoon paprika
1 teaspoon dried chopped onion *or*
    1 tablespoon minced fresh onion

In a small bowl or cup, combine all ingredients. Mix well. Add to the browned meat and ¾ cup of water. Simmer to allow flavors to blend.

MACARONI AND CHEESE–STYLE SAUCE, DAIRY-FREE

Makes approximately 1 1/2 cups

Here is a dairy-free, creamy sauce to substitute for traditional cheese sauce. The navy beans add body; the turmeric adds yellow color; the oil adds a creamy mouth-feel, and the nutritional yeast adds a complexity to the flavor. Very pleasant.

  1 cup rice milk
  2 tablespoons potato starch
  1 teaspoon garlic salt
  ½ teaspoon onion powder
  ¼ teaspoon turmeric
  ¼ cup canola oil
  ¼ cup canned navy beans (drained)
  1 tablespoon nutritional yeast (optional)

Combine all ingredients except for the beans and the yeast in a microwave-safe bowl. Mix well. Microwave on high for approximately 1½ to 2 minutes until thick. Stir once during microwaving. Pour the sauce into a blender. Add the beans and yeast (if desired). Process on high until the mixture is smooth. Serve hot over gluten-free pasta.

PIZZA SAUCE

Makes approximately 3½ cups

Tomato puree is the perfect consistency for use in pizza sauce. When you purchase the tomato puree, try to find one with no extra spices or salt. I like to use extra virgin olive oil for its great flavor in this recipe.

  one 28-ounce can tomato puree
  2 tablespoons olive oil
  2 teaspoons dried oregano or Italian seasoning
  2 teaspoons garlic salt

In a medium saucepan, combine all ingredients. Simmer at a near boil for 15 minutes for flavors to blend.

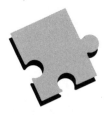

Crackers and Snacks

SORGHUM CRACKERS

Makes approximately 60 one-inch-square crackers

These are light and crispy whole-grain crackers, similar to Wheat Thins.

½ cup trans fat–free shortening
1 teaspoon apple cider vinegar
1½ cups sorghum flour, 200 grams
½ teaspoon baking soda
½ teaspoon salt
1½ teaspoon xanthan gum
½ cup plain lowfat dairy-free yogurt

Topping:
salt (flaky sea salt is nice)

Preheat the oven to 375°F. Lightly grease a baking sheet.

In a medium-sized bowl, combine all ingredients except yogurt. Beat until fine crumbs form. Add the yogurt and beat until dough comes together.

Pat out dough onto a baking sheet as thinly as possible (⅛-inch thick or less). Use a sharp knife to cut a grid pattern across dough to form squares. Use a fork to pierce holes throughout the tops of crackers. Sprinkle tops with salt. Bake for approximately 10 to 12 minutes, until tops are lightly browned.

CLUB-STYLE CRACKERS

Makes approximately 24

These crackers are softly crisp. They have an understated whole grain flavor. A small amount of turmeric may be added for yellow coloring if desired.

⅓ cup trans fat-free shortening
1 teaspoon apple cider vinegar
¾ cup brown rice flour, 95 grams
¾ cup sorghum flour, 100 grams
½ teaspoon baking soda
½ teaspoon salt
1 teaspoon xanthan gum
¼ cup apple juice

Topping:
　salt

Preheat the oven to 375 °F. Lightly grease a cookie sheet.

In a medium-size bowl, combine all ingredients, except the apple juice. Beat until fine crumbs form. Add the apple juice and mix well. Batter will barely come together as a dough.

Press dough to ⅛-inch (or less) thickness in the shape of a traditional crackers, approximately 2 inches square. Use a pizza cutter to make cracker squares. Remove "straggler" dough and press out again to form more crackers. Use fork to pierce holes throughout the tops of the crackers. Sprinkle tops with salt.

Bake for approximately 12 minutes, until the top is nicely browned. If taken out too soon, the cracker will remain soft (but pleasant) instead of crisping.

GRAHAM CRACKER–STYLE COOKIES

Makes 9 or 10 four-part cookies

These cookies are so good! And easy to make, too! A traditional graham cracker measures approximately 5 inches by 2¼ inches. Yours can, too!

⅓ cup trans fat-free shortening
½ cup honey
1 tablespoon unsulphured molasses
¾ cup brown rice flour, 95 grams
¾ cup sorghum flour, 100 grams
½ teaspoon baking soda
½ teaspoon salt
1 teaspoon xanthan gum

Preheat the oven to 375 °F. Lightly grease a cookie sheet.

In a medium-size bowl, combine shortening, honey, and molasses. Beat well. Add the remaining ingredients and beat well. Batter will be thick and pasty.

Place one rounded tablespoon of dough onto the prepared pan. Spread to ⅛-inch (or less) thickness in the shape of a traditional graham cracker. (Moistened fingertips make this task easier.) Use a pizza cutter to make clean edges and indentations for break areas of the cracker. Use a fork to pierce holes throughout the top of the cookie.

Bake for approximately 13 minutes, until the top is nicely browned. If taken out too soon, cookie will remain bendable instead of crisping.

Use a pizza cutter to remove the excess cookie from the edges. Discard or snack on these little strips. Move the cookies to a cooling rack to cool completely. Cookies will harden as they cool.

SOFT PRETZELS

Makes 4 to 6 soft pretzels or 20 to 25 short pretzel sticks

Be sure to bake these pretzels to a full golden-brown color in order to achieve a nice exterior texture. I prefer the flavor at room temperature, but hot from the oven is nice, too.

    3 egg whites
    1 tablespoon canola oil
    ½ cup unsweetened applesauce
    ¼ cup apple juice
    1 cup brown rice flour, 125 grams
    2 teaspoons Rumford baking powder
    1 teaspoon baking soda
    ½ teaspoon salt
    1⅛ teaspoons xanthan gum
    1 tablespoon apple cider vinegar

Topping:
    water for spraying
    coarse salt

Preheat oven to 375 °F. Lightly grease a baking sheet.

In a medium-size bowl, beat the egg whites until very frothy. Add the remaining ingredients. Mix well. Batter will be light and pillowy. Place the dough into a large, square plastic bag. Snip one corner off the bottom edge of the bag, approximately ½ inch wide.

Pipe the shape of soft pretzel by first imagining the face of a clock. Start at 10 o'clock, moving in a straight line to 5 o'clock, then arching up and around the face of the clock counterclockwise all the way back to 7 o'clock, then drawing a straight line up to 2 o'clock. Or simply pipe out some pretzel sticks.

Spray the pretzel shapes with salt water, then sprinkle with salt, and place in the oven. Bake for approximately 15 to 20 minutes until very golden brown in color. Remove from oven.

TORTILLA CHIPS

Serves 12

Mildly flavored chips.

6 tortillas (from recipe on page 157)

¼ teaspoon salt
2 cups canola oil

Cut tortillas into wedges.

Over high heat, heat oil to 360 °F. Fry the wedges until lightly browned. Drain on paper towels and sprinkle lightly with salt.

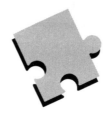

Everyday Meals

CHICKEN NUGGETS (BAKED)

Serves 4

Although I use gluten-free crispy rice–style cereal to make the coating for these nuggets, another gluten-free plain cereal (such as Rice Chex—gluten-free as of this writing) may be used in its place. Double-dipping in the egg wash assures a light, crisp coating.

1 pound boneless chicken breast or "tenders"

Breading:
2 cups gluten-free crispy rice–style cereal
½ teaspoon salt
½ teaspoon pepper (optional)
1 egg (omega-3 enriched)
2 tablespoons water
½ cup brown rice flour

Preheat oven to 375 °F. Spray the baking sheet lightly with nonstick spray.
　　Cut chicken into small serving-size pieces.

Crush cereal to a fine texture. (You may wish to place the cereal in zip-type bag and crush with a rolling pin.) Cereal should yield nearly ¾ cups of crumbs. Place cereal crumbs onto a plate. Add salt and stir. Set aside.

In a small bowl, combine the egg and water. Beat well to form an egg wash—the color of the mixture should be uniform, not streaky. Place the brown rice flour on a separate plate.

Dip chicken pieces into the egg wash, then immediately dip them into the brown rice flour. Dip again into the egg wash and finally into the crumb mixture. Place on a prepared pan. Continue until all the chicken is coated.

Bake for approximately 15 to 20 minutes, depending upon the size of the nuggets. The chicken should be cooked through, with no pink remaining.

CHICKEN NUGGETS (FRIED)

Serves 4

Chicken nuggets are best fried in a deeper amount of oil to ensure that the nuggets do not rest (and stick) to the bottom of the pan. I like to use a fork to hold the nugget away from the sides of the pan for the first few moments of frying.

1 pound boneless chicken breast or "tenders"

Batter:
- ½ cup brown rice flour, 65 grams
- ¼ cup sorghum flour, 35 grams
- ½ teaspoon salt
- ½ teaspoon baking powder
- ¼ teaspoon xanthan gum
- 1 cup apple juice

For frying: 2 cups canola oil

Cut chicken into small serving-size pieces. Heat oil in small pan to 370 °F.

Combine batter ingredients in a small bowl. Dip chicken into the batter and fry in hot oil for 4 to 7 minutes, depending upon the size of the nuggets. The chicken should be cooked through, with no pink remaining.

The outer coating will be golden brown.

CRISPY FISH STICKS

Serves 4 to 6

These fish sticks will best any traditional, frozen fish stick. Leave fillets whole if you need faster preparation time.

4 Tilapia fish fillets or other firm, white fish
Breading:
3 cups gluten-free crispy rice–style cereal
¼ cup canola oil
½ teaspoon salt
½ teaspoon pepper (optional)

Preheat oven to 400 °F. Spray baking sheet lightly with nonstick spray.

Cut fish into strips. Set aside.

Place cereal, salt, and pepper in zip-type bag. Crush into a fine texture. Cereal should yield approximately 1 cup of crumbs. Place crumbs onto a plate. Set aside.

Place oil in a small bowl. Dip fish sticks first into the oil, then immediately roll them in the crumbs. Place on a prepared pan. Continue until all fish sticks are coated.

Bake for approximately 15 minutes until fish is cooked through and no longer opaque.

CRISPY OVEN-BAKED CHICKEN PIECES

Makes 8 pieces

To save the hassle of making (or the cost of buying) gluten-free bread crumbs, this recipe uses crushed gluten-free cereal.

  1 whole chicken, cut into pieces, about 4 ½ pounds
  2 cups gluten-free rice cereal
  ¼ teaspoon salt
  ¼ teaspoon black pepper
  ¼ teaspoon paprika

Preheat oven to 400 °F. Lightly grease an 8½ x 13 inch baking pan.

Rinse chicken and place in pan. Place rice cereal, salt, pepper, and paprika in a zip-type bag and crush into fine crumbs. Sprinkle crumbs evenly over top of chicken pieces. Or, if preferred, chicken may be placed into the bag and shaken to coat all over.

Bake for 60 minutes until chicken is cooked through and no pink remains.

SPAGHETTI AND MEATBALLS

Using the vegetable puree in this sauce is a great way to increase the nutritional value in this kid-favorite dish. Substitute 6 ounces of any baby-food vegetable (puree style) or finely diced fresh vegetables in its place.

For Sauce:

Makes approximately 4 cups

> one 28-ounce can crushed tomatoes
> ¾ cup vegetable puree (page 210)
> 1 small onion, peeled and finely diced
> 2 tablespoons olive oil
> 2 teaspoons dried oregano or Italian seasoning
> 1 teaspoon garlic salt
> ½ teaspoon sea salt
> 1 teaspoon honey (optional)

In medium saucepan, combine all the ingredients. Simmer at a near boil for 15 minutes for flavors to blend. Sauce may be pureed in blender if a smoother texture is desired.

For Meatballs:

Makes 20 to 25 one-inch meatballs

> ½ pound lean ground beef
> ½ pound ground pork
> ½ small onion, peeled and minced
> 1 teaspoon sea salt
> 1 teaspoon dried oregano or Italian seasoning
> ½ teaspoon black pepper
> 1 tablespoon canola oil

In medium-size bowl, combine all ingredients, except oil. Gently mix together until well blended. Shape into one-inch size round meatballs.

Over medium heat, place oil in a large pan. Add meatballs and cook until done, approximately 7 to 10 minutes. No pink should remain. Add to the sauce or place on top of the spaghetti as desired.

For Spaghetti:

Serves 4

> one 12-ounce package gluten-free spaghetti or other
>   gluten-free pasta

Cook according to package directions. Top with sauce and meatballs.

SAUSAGE

Makes 1 pound

Fresh sausage tastes a little bit different from store-purchased sausage, but I think you will really enjoy it! Compared to most commercial brands, I believe you will find this version leaner and lighter in color. These differences arise from use of leaner, freshly ground pork and different cuts of pork. If you have time, mix the sausage up ahead of time so flavors have time to blend.

> 1 pound ground pork
> 1 tablespoon canola oil
> 1 tablespoon apple juice
> ¾ teaspoon salt
> 1 tablespoon rubbed or dried sage
> 1½ teaspoons dried thyme
> 1 teaspoon black pepper
> 1 teaspoon fennel seed
> 1 teaspoon honey

Combine all ingredients in a mixing bowl. Mix very well. Use as you would any prepared sausage.

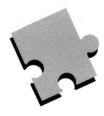

Microwave Baking

INDIVIDUAL CHOCOLATE CAKE

Makes 2 small layers

Like the yellow cake, this recipe makes two tiny layers. Although it poofs a great deal during cooking, it settles flat while cooling.

1 egg (omega-3 enriched)
2 tablespoons canola oil
3 tablespoons applesauce
tiny pinch of salt
1 tablespoon brown rice flour
1 tablespoon sorghum flour
1 tablespoon cocoa
⅛ teaspoon baking soda
1 tablespoon honey
¼ teaspoon vanilla

In a small bowl or cup, briefly stir the egg to form little bubbles. Add the remaining ingredients and mix well. Spray two ramekins (or other microwave-safe bowl that holds at least ¾ cup) with nonstick spray. Pour batter into the ramekins. Microwave on high for two minutes. Gently remove from dishes and allow to cool.

INDIVIDUAL CHOCOLATE CHIP MUFFINS

Makes 2

This recipe makes two muffins with a light and moist texture. These muffins do not dome during cooking. Enjoy!

1 egg (omega-3 enriched)
2 tablespoons canola oil
2 tablespoons applesauce
tiny pinch of salt
2 tablespoons brown rice flour
1 tablespoon sorghum flour
¼ teaspoon baking powder
⅛ teaspoon baking soda
¼ teaspoon xanthan gum
1 tablespoon honey
¼ teaspoon vanilla
3 tablespoons GFCF semisweet chocolate chips,
    finely chopped

In a small bowl or cup, briefly stir the egg to form little bubbles. Add the remaining ingredients, except chips, and mix well. Fold in the chips. Spray two ramekins (or other microwave-safe bowl that holds at least ¾ cup) with nonstick spray. Pour batter into the ramekins. Microwave on high for two minutes. Gently remove from dishes and allow to cool.

INDIVIDUAL ENGLISH MUFFIN

Makes 1

Make this English muffin and then toast it for a quick and tasty breakfast treat.

1 egg white
2 teaspoons canola oil
1 tablespoon applesauce
tiny pinch of salt
2 tablespoons brown rice flour

1 tablespoon sorghum flour
½ teaspoon Rumford baking powder
⅛ teaspoon baking soda
¼ teaspoon honey

In a small bowl or cup, briefly stir the egg white to form little bubbles. Add the remaining ingredients and mix well. Spray a one-cup ramekin (or other microwave-safe bowl) with nonstick spray. Spread batter into the ramekin. Microwave on high for one minute. Gently remove from the dish and allow to cool. Split in half and toast before serving.

INDIVIDUAL FRUIT COBBLER

Serves 1

This recipe makes a single cobbler, although you may wish to make more. Frozen mixed berries are very nice in this dish.

For fruit layer:
   ½ cup chopped frozen fruit
   1 tablespoon honey

For top layer:
   2 tablespoons brown rice flour
   1 tablespoon sorghum flour
   1 tablespoon trans fat-free shortening
   ¼ teaspoon baking powder
   ¼ teaspoon xanthan gum
   ¼ teaspoon vanilla
   1 tablespoon honey

Lightly grease two ramekins (or other microwave-safe bowls). Place fruit and honey in the ramekins. Microwave on high for 45 seconds.

In small bowl or cup, mix all ingredients for the top layer. Mix well. Break dough pieces over the fruit. Microwave on high for 1 minute.

INDIVIDUAL ROLLS

Makes 1

Inspired by a recipe for Very Low-Carb Hamburger Bun at www.recipezaar.com/229625, this roll takes just minutes from start to finish. A standard 3½ inch ramekin was used for cooking, but any small microwave-safe bowl should do just fine. This roll is moist and best at room temperature.

1 egg white
1 tablespoon canola oil
2 tablespoons applesauce
tiny pinch of salt
2 tablespoons brown rice flour

1 tablespoon sorghum flour
½ teaspoon baking powder
small pinch of baking soda
pinch of flaxseed meal (optional)

In a small bowl or cup, briefly stir the egg white to form little bubbles. Add the remaining ingredients and mix well. Spray a ramekin (or other microwave-safe bowl) with nonstick spray. Spread batter into the ramekin. Top with flaxseed meal (for aesthetics) if desired. Microwave on high for one minute. Gently remove from dish and allow to cool.

INDIVIDUAL YELLOW CAKE

Makes 2 small layers

This recipe makes two layers of a really small cake. It is ready in just minutes in the microwave.

1 egg (omega-3 enriched)
2 tablespoons canola oil
3 tablespoons applesauce
tiny pinch of salt
2 tablespoons brown rice flour
1 tablespoon sorghum flour
¼ teaspoon baking powder
1 tablespoon honey
¼ teaspoon vanilla

In a small bowl or cup, briefly stir the egg to form little bubbles. Add the remaining ingredients and mix well. Spray two ramekins (or other microwave-safe bowl that holds at least ¾ cup) with nonstick spray. Pour batter into the ramekins. Microwave on high for two minutes. Gently remove from dishes and allow to cool.

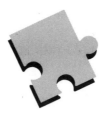

Soups

CHICKEN SOUP

Makes approximately 10 cups

To avoid use of bouillon cubes or prepackaged stock, this recipe uses a super-fast stock of its own. Tinkyada makes a nice spaghetti-style pasta that works well in this soup. Any gluten-free pasta or rice may be substituted as desired.

2 tablespoons canola or olive oil
3 carrots, washed (do not peel)
1 large onion, washed (do not peel)
4 leg-and-thigh chicken quarters,
   approximately 2 ½ pounds
10 cups hot water (filtered)
1 medium onion, peeled,
   then finely diced

1 tablespoon dried parsley (optional)
½ teaspoon black pepper (optional)
2 teaspoons sea salt
8 ounces Tinkyada spaghetti-style
   pasta, broken in pieces

Place the oil in a large pot. Turn heat to high. Cut the carrots in half and add to the pot. Cut the onion in quarters and add to the pot. Add the chicken pieces. Cook, turning the chicken frequently until it browns, approximately 8 minutes.

Carefully add 10 cups of hot water to the pot. Cover and cook until the chicken is very tender (approximately 15 minutes after the water boils). Remove all but the broth from the pot. Discard the cooked carrots and onions. Debone the chicken and cut into small pieces. Add the deboned chicken to the broth.

Add finely diced onion, parsley, salt, and pasta to the broth. Cook uncovered (at a slow boil) until the pasta is tender (approximately 15 minutes for Tinkyada). If flavor is too mild, continue cooking to allow the broth to reduce.

TOMATO SOUP

Makes approximately 4 cups

This recipe is fashioned after Campbell's tomato soup, which contains both high fructose corn syrup and wheat flour (at the time of writing). It takes just a few minutes to make this family favorite. For a richer flavor, 1 tablespoon oil plus rice milk may be substituted equally for all or part of the water.

    one 6-ounce can tomato paste
    four 6-ounce cans water (filtered)
    ½ teaspoon garlic salt
    ½ teaspoon sea salt
    ¼ teaspoon paprika
    1 tablespoon honey (or ¼ teaspoon stevia)

In a medium saucepan, combine all ingredients. Stir well. Simmer for several minutes for the flavors to blend. Serve hot.

VEGETABLE SOUP

Makes 9 cups

This vegetarian vegetable soup is very flavorful. Please note that I use canned crushed or diced tomatoes that have only tomatoes listed on the ingredient panel. Rienzi is a nice Italian brand. The soup comes together in minutes. If your canned tomatoes have salt as an ingredient, you will want to reduce the amount of salt called for in this recipe. Add small pieces of cooked beef, chicken, or even crabmeat if desired.

    2 tablespoons oil (olive oil preferred)
    1 small onion, peeled and diced
    one 28-ounce can crushed or diced tomatoes, 800 grams
    one 28-ounce can water (3 ½ cups) (filtered)
    1 small red potato, cut in half, then thinly sliced
    1 pound mixed frozen vegetables
    1 teaspoon sea salt
    2 teaspoons Old Bay (or creole) seasoning

Over medium heat, place the oil and onion in a medium to large saucepan. Cook until the onion softens. Add the remaining ingredients, including juice from the tomatoes. Turn heat down to a low boil. Cook uncovered until all the vegetables are very tender, approximately 20 minutes.

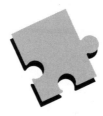

Vegetables and Sides

BAKED VEGETABLE STICKS

Serves 2

These veggies are oven-roasted to tender-crisp. Because the shape is similar to that of French fries, they may be more readily welcomed into the diet. Turning the sticks during baking will make for a more uniform texture.

4 carrots, 12 ounces *or*
1 large russet potato, 10 ounces *or*
   1 large sweet potato, 10 ounces *or*
   2 small to medium zucchini squash, 12 ounces
up to 1 tablespoon canola oil
⅛ teaspoon salt
Preheat oven to 400 °F.
Lightly grease a baking sheet.

For carrots: Wash and peel. Cut into French fry shape, approximately ¼ inch thick. Toss in oil and place on a prepared baking sheet. Sprinkle lightly with salt and bake for approximately 20 to 25 minutes until tender-crisp.

For potato: Wash and peel. Cut into French fry shape, approximately ¼ inch thick. Toss in oil and place on a prepared baking sheet. Sprinkle lightly with salt and bake for approximately 30 minutes until tender-crisp.

For sweet potato: Wash and peel. Cut into French fry shape, approximately ¼ inch thick. Toss in oil and place on a prepared baking sheet. Sprinkle lightly with salt and bake for approximately 15 to 20 minutes until tender-crisp.

For zucchini squash: Wash, but do not peel. Cut into French fry shape, approximately ¼ inch thick. Toss in oil and place on a prepared baking sheet. Sprinkle with salt and bake for approximately 8 to 9 minutes until tender-crisp.

MASHED POTATOES

Serves 4

Without dairy, mashed potatoes lack creaminess. Oil is added to this recipe to offset this characteristic.

>   **1 pound of russet or Yukon gold potatoes**
>   **½ cup rice milk**
>   **2 teaspoons canola oil**
>   **¼ teaspoon sea salt**

Wash, peel, and chop potatoes into large chunks. Place in a saucepan and cover with water. Over medium heat, boil for approximately 10 to 15 minutes until potatoes are very tender. Drain potatoes and return them to the pan or mixing bowl. Add milk, oil, and salt. Beat until light and creamy.

MASHED SWEET POTATOES

Serves 4

If your child likes mashed potatoes, this recipe may be good for introducing a new food in a familiar form. Lightly sweetened by the apple juice, they are tasty.

> **1 pound of sweet potatoes or yams**
> **½ cup apple juice**
> **pinch of sea salt**

Wash, peel, and chop sweet potatoes into large chunks. Place in a large saucepan and cover with water. Over medium heat, boil for approximately 10 to 15 minutes, until potatoes are very tender. Drain potatoes and return to the pan or mixing bowl. Add juice and salt. Beat until light and creamy.

QUICK FRENCH FRIES

Serves 2

Although it is traditional to twice-fry fries to achieve that delicious crispness, this recipe has been shortcut to do the initial cooking in the microwave. The fries are crisp outside and tender inside, just as they should be.

> **1 large russet potato, 10 ounces**
> **2 cups canola oil (not olive)**
> **⅛ teaspoon salt**

Pierce potato with a fork or a knife. Microwave on high for approximately 3 minutes to partially cook the potato. Cool for several minutes. Cut into ¼ inch thick-fries.

   Heat oil in frying pan to 370 °F. (A fry will sizzle when added to the pan.) Add cut fries and cook them until they are nicely browned and cooked through, approximately 10 minutes. Remove and drain on paper towels. Sprinkle lightly with salt.

SPANISH RICE

Serves 5 to 6

This recipe is so easy, you may wonder why you bothered with mixes in the first place! This was preferred over the boxed competitor by our testers.

3 cups water (filtered)
1½ cups rice
1 tablespoon canola oil
2 plum tomatoes, finely chopped
½ small onion, finely chopped
¼ small red or green bell pepper, finely chopped
1½ teaspoons paprika
1 teaspoon garlic salt
1½ teaspoons chili powder
½ teaspoon salt

In medium saucepan, combine all ingredients. Stir well and bring to a boil. Cover and simmer for approximately 15 minutes until rice is tender and water is absorbed. If you prefer softer rice, add an additional ⅓ cup of water and cover with lid for several minutes.

VEGETABLE PUREE

Makes approximately 3 cups

Use this simple puree in the spaghetti and meatballs recipe (page 196) or add to soups and other sauces to increase nutritional value. A vegetable puree can be made from nearly any vegetable. Experiment with whatever is in season.

one 16-ounce package frozen mixed vegetables
1 cup water (filtered)

Place vegetables and water in a medium-size saucepan. Cook over high heat (covered) until vegetables are very tender, approximately 5 minutes after boiling.

Place in a blender and puree until very smooth. Pulsing the blender helps to move the cooked vegetables during the process. Add additional water (as little as possible) if needed to puree.

PART III
NUTRITIONAL INFORMATION

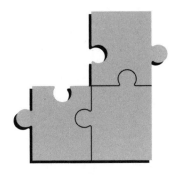

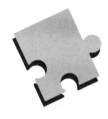

APPENDIX 1

Choosing a Registered Dietitian

WHAT IS A REGISTERED DIETITIAN (RD)?

A registered dietitian is a food and nutrition expert who provides her clients with reliable, objective nutrition information, helps them separate fact from fiction, and translates the latest scientific findings into understandable nutrition information. A registered dietitian offers Medical Nutrition Therapy (MNT), in which she makes a comprehensive assessment of your child's nutritional status by analyzing his medical and diet history, laboratory test results, weight and growth measurements, and feeding skills. Using this information, an RD will develop an individualized nutrition treatment plan for your child, provide nutrition counseling, nutrition-care coordination, and will monitor his progress.

WHAT TYPE OF EDUCATION AND TRAINING DOES AN RD RECEIVE?

In order to be considered a nationally accredited registered dietitian, RDs must complete a minimum of a bachelor's degree in dietetics, foods and nutrition, or a related area at an accredited U.S. college or university. They must also complete a supervised clinical experience of at least six to twelve months in length and pass a national examination.

In addition, many states have regulatory laws governing dietitians. Today, approximately forty-six states have laws that regulate dietitians or nutritionists through licensure, certification, or registration. For information on your state's regulations, check with the Commission of Dietetic Registration (CDR), the credentialing agency for the American Dietetic Association, at www.cdrnet.org/certifications/licensure.

WHAT IS THE DIFFERENCE BETWEEN A REGISTERED DIETITIAN AND A NUTRITIONIST?

The terms *dietitian* and *nutritionist* are often used interchangeably, but there's a big difference between the two that you need to be aware of. In the United States, the term *dietitian* is legally protected, and an individual can't use the title "dietitian" unless she has met the specific educational and experiential requirements and passed the national registration exam. On the other hand, the term *nutritionist* is *not* legally protected in the United States. Some, but not all, states do offer some form of legal protection for the term *nutritionist*. Therefore, it's important to remember that a "nutritionist" may not actually have any education, training, or experience in foods and nutrition. If you're seeking the counsel of a "nutritionist," be sure to ask if she's a registered dietitian and/or a licensed or certified dietitian or nutritionist within her state.

HOW DO I FIND A REGISTERED DIETITIAN?

There are several ways to locate an RD. Here are a few suggestions:

1. Contact the American Dietetic Association (ADA) at www.eatright.org. Click on the "Find a Nutrition Professional" link, then click on the "Find a Nutrition Professional Consumer Search" link. You'll be directed to enter your area code and state to get a listing of registered dietitians in your community.

2. Contact your state dietetic association. Most state dietetic association Web sites have a link called "Find a Dietitian" for consumers looking for a list of registered dietitians in their community.

3. Contact the Nutrition in Complementary Care (NCC), a dietary practice group of the American Dietetic Association. The NCC is a group of registered dietitians interested in alternative therapies and dietary supplements, and you can reach them at www.complementarynutrition.org. Just enter your state under "Find-A-Comp Care" and you'll get a list of registered dietitians in your state interested in complementary nutrition care.

4. If your child is under the age of three and has a developmental disability or delay, he may qualify to receive services from a statewide program called Early Childhood Intervention (ECI). A registered dietitian is part of the team of service providers in an ECI Program.

HOW DO I CHOOSE THE RIGHT REGISTERED DIETITIAN FOR MY CHILD?

Finding a registered dietitian is not difficult, but finding the *right* dietitian for your child can be a challenge. Just like any other healthcare professional, registered dietitians have specific areas of expertise and personal interest. Not all registered dietitians have experience in providing services to children with autism and other related disorders. It's important to find a dietitian who can meet your child's unique dietary needs. Once you have a list of registered dietitians in your community, I suggest you narrow the list down by asking each dietitian the following questions:

- What type of training and experience do you have working with children with autism and related disorders such as Asperger's, PDD, and ADHD?
- Are you comfortable recommending nutritional supplements, herbs, and nutraceuticals?
- Are you interested in complementary and alternative medicine?
- Are you a member of the Nutrition in Complementary Care (NCC) dietary practice group of the American Dietetic Association?
- If you have experience with providing nutrition therapy to children with other developmental disabilities, but not autism, are you willing to learn?

If you have trouble finding the right registered dietitian for your child in your local community, please don't give up. Expand your search to neighboring communities until you find the right match.

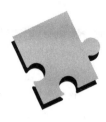

APPENDIX 2

The Best Dietary Sources for Protein, Fiber, and Calcium

PROTEIN		
Food	**Serving Size**	**(grams)**
Beans (cooked)		
Beans (black, kidney, lima, navy, pinto)	1 cup	15
Beans, white	1 cup	17
Chickpeas (garbanzo beans)	1 cup	15
Beef (cooked)		
Beef, retail cuts, all grades	3 ounces	22
Frankfurter, beef (8 per 1 pound)	1 each	6
Ground beef	3 ounces	22
Ribs	3 ounces	19
Cheese		
Cheese, cheddar	1 ounce	7
Cheese, mozzarella	1 ounce	6
Cheese, Swiss	1 ounce	8
Cheese, goat	1 ounce	5
Cheese, cottage, creamed	1 cup	26
Cheese, processed, American	1 slice (¾ oz)	5

Egg

Egg, fresh, whole	1 large	6
Egg substitute, powder	¾ ounce	11

Fish (cooked)

Cod, Atlantic	3 ounces	19
Salmon, Atlantic, wild	3 ounces	22
Salmon, Atlantic, farmed	3 ounces	19
Tuna, light, canned in oil	3 ounces	25
Tuna, light, canned in water	3 ounces	22
Tuna, white, canned in oil	3 ounces	23
Tuna, white, canned in water	3 ounces	20
White, mixed species	3 ounces	21
Shrimp, breaded & fried	4 large	6

Milk

Milk, whole	1 cup	8
Milk, nonfat (skim or fat free)	1 cup	8
Milk, low fat, 1% milk fat	1 cup	8
Milk, reduced fat, 2% milk fat	1 cup	8
Milk, dry powder, nonfat	¼ cup	11

Nuts/Seeds

Almonds, raw	1 cup	30
Almonds	1 ounce (23 each)	6
Cashews, dry roasted	1 cup	21
Cashews	1 ounce	4
Mixed nuts with peanuts, dry roasted	1 cup	24
Mixed nuts	1 ounce	5
Peanuts, all types, dry roasted	1 cup	35
Peanuts	1 ounce	7
Pecans, halves	1 cup	10
Pecans	1 ounce (19 halves)	3
Pine nuts	1 cup	19
Pine nuts	1 ounce (167 kernels)	4
Pistachios, raw	1 cup	25

PROTEIN *(Continued)*

Food	Serving Size	(grams)
Nuts/Seeds (cont.)		
Pistachios	1 ounce (49 kernels)	6
Pumpkin & squash seeds, roasted	1 cup	31
Pumpkin & squash seeds	1 ounce	9
Sunflower seeds, kernels, roasted	1 cup, hulled	25
Sunflower seeds	1 ounce	6
Walnuts	1 cup (50 halves)	15
Walnuts	1 ounce (14 halves)	4
Peanut Butter		
Peanut butter, chunk & smooth style	1 Tbsp	4
Pork (cooked)		
Bacon	1 slice	3
Chop, loin	3 ounces	22
Frankfurter, pork	1 each	10
Ham	3 ounces	23
Ribs, country-style	3 ounces	20
Roast, top loin	3 ounces	23
Poultry (cooked)		
Chicken breast	1/2 breast	29
Chicken drumstick	1 each	14
Chicken thigh	1 each	16
Chicken wing	1 each	9
Frankfurt, chicken	1 each	7
Chicken nuggets, fast food	4 pieces	10
Chicken tenders, fast food	4 pieces	11
Cornish hen	½ bird	29
Turkey, all classes, dark meat	1 cup	39
Turkey, all classes, light meat	1 cup	40
Turkey, bacon	1 ounce	5
Turkey, ground	3 ounces	17

Soy

Soybean, curd cheese	1 cup	28
Soybeans, mature seed, roasted	1 cup	61
Soy burger, veggie burger	1 patty	11
Soymilk, original, vanilla and chocolate (fortified with calcium, vitamins A and D)	1 cup	6
Tofu, raw, firm	1 cup	40

Yogurt

Yogurt, plain, whole milk	1 cup	9
Yogurt, plain, low fat	1 cup	12
Yogurt, plain, skim milk	1 cup	14
Yogurt, fruit variety, nonfat	1 cup	11
Yogurt, tofu	1 cup	9

Baby Food Meats (Strained)

Beef	2½ ounce jar	9
Chicken	2½ ounce jar	10
Ham	2½ ounce jar	8
Lamb	2½ ounce jar	10
Turkey	2½ ounce jar	8

Misc.

Pizza, frozen, cheese topping	1 slice	8
Pizza, fast food chain, cheese topping	1 slice	12
Macaroni and cheese	1 cup	11

FIBER

Food	Serving Size	(grams)
Beans/Peas (cooked)		
Beans, Navy	1 cup	19
Beans, Pinto	1 cup	15
Beans, Black	1 cup	15
Beans, Lima	1 cup	13

(Continues)

FIBER *(Continued)*

Food	Serving Size	(grams)
Beans/Peas (cooked) (cont.)		
Garbanzo beans	1 cup	13
Beans, white	1 cup	11
Peas, split	1 cup	16
Soy		
Soybeans, mature seeds, roasted	1 cup	30
Nuts/Seeds		
Almonds	1 cup	19
Mixed nuts with peanuts	1 cup	12
Peanuts	1 cup	12
Sunflower seeds, dry roasted	1 cup, hulled	14
Whole Grains		
Bread, whole wheat	1 slice	1
Bread, multi-grain	1 slice	2
Bread, pita, whole wheat	1 small	2
Bread, rye	1 slice	2
Brown rice	1 cup	4
Vegetables		
Broccoli	1 cup	2
Brussels sprouts	1 cup	6
Corn, sweet, canned	1 cup	3
Carrot, raw	1 medium	2
Green beans, canned	1 cup	4
Potato, baked, with skin	1 medium	4
Tomato paste	½ cup	5
Turnip greens, frozen	1 cup	6
Fruits (raw)		
Apple, with skin	1 medium	4
Banana	1 medium	3

Orange	1 each	3
Peach	1 medium	2
Pear	1 medium	6
Raisin	1 small box (1.5 oz)	2
Strawberries	1 cup	3

Snack

Popcorn, air popped	1 cup	1

CALCIUM

Food	Serving Size	(mg)
Milk, whole	1 cup	276
Milk, dry powder, nonfat	¼ cup	377
Soymilk (fortified with calcium)	1 cup	199
Yogurt, plain, whole milk	1 cup	296
Cheese, cheddar	1 ounce	204
Cheese, mozzarella	1 ounce	143
Cheese, Swiss	1 ounce	224
Cheese, goat	1 ounce	40
Cheese, cottage, creamed	1 cup	126
Cheese, processed, American	1 slice (¾ oz)	144
Kraft macaroni and cheese	1 cup	92
Tofu, raw, regular	½ cup	434
Tofu, yogurt	1 cup	309
Orange juice (fortified with calcium)	1 cup	300
Rice Dream, non-dairy beverage	1 cup	300
Vance's Dari Free	1 cup	240

Source: USDA, Agricultural Research Service, Nutrient Data Laboratory

Appendix 3

RDA or AI and UL for Vitamins and Minerals

Dietary Reference Intakes (DRIs): Recommended Intakes for Individuals, Vitamins

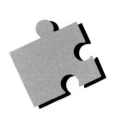

Life Stage Group	Vit.A (µg/d)[a]	Vit.C (mg/d)	Vit.D (µg/d)[b,c]	Vit.E (mg/d)[d]	Vit.K (µg/d)	Thiamin (mg/d)	Riboflavin (mg/d)	Niacin (mg/d)[e]	Vit.B6 (mg/d)	Folate (µg/d)[f]	Vit.B12 (µg/d)	Pantothenic Acid (mg/d)	Biotin (µg/d)	Choline[g] (mg/d)
Children														
1–3 y	300	15	5*	6	30*	0.5	0.5	6	0.5	150	0.9	2*	8*	200*
4–8 y	400	25	5*	7	55*	0.6	0.6	8	0.6	200	1.2	3*	12*	250*
Males														
9–13 y	600	45	5*	11	60*	0.9	0.9	12	1.0	300	1.8	4*	20*	375*
14–18 y	900	75	5*	15	75*	1.2	1.3	16	1.3	400	2.4	5*	25*	550*
19–50 y	900	90	5*	15	120*	1.2	1.3	16	1.3	400	2.4	5*	30*	550*

Females

9–13 y	**600**	**45**	5*	**11**	60*	**0.9**	**0.9**	**12**	**1.0**	**300**	**1.8**	4*	20*	375*
14–18 y	**700**	**65**	5*	**15**	75*	**1.0**	**1.0**	**14**	**1.2**	**400**	**2.4**	5*	25*	400*
19–50 y	**700**	**75**	5*	**15**	90*	**1.1**	**1.1**	**14**	**1.3**	**400**	**2.4**	5*	30*	425*

Recommended Dietary Allowances (RDAs) are in **bold type**, and Adequate Intakes (AIs) are in ordinary type followed by an asterisk (*).

[a] As retinol activity equivalents (RAEs), 1 RAE = 1 μg retinol, 12 μg ß-carotene, 24 μg α-carotene, or 24 μg ß-cryptoxanthin. The RAE for dietary provitamin A carotenoids is twofold greater than retinol equivalents (RE), whereas the RAE for preformed vitamin A is the same as RE.

[b] As cholecalciferol, 1 μg cholecalciferol = 40 IU vitamin D.

[c] In the absence of adequate exposure to sunlight.

[d] As α-tocopherol, α-Tocopherol includes *RRR*-α-tocopherol, the only form of α-tocopherol that occurs naturally in foods, and the 2R-stereoisomeric forms of α-tocopherol (*RRR*-, *RSR*-, *RRS*-, and *RSS*-α-tocopherol) that occur in fortified foods and supplements. It does not include the 2S-stereoisomeric forms of α-tocopherol (*SRR*-, *SSR*-, *SRS*-, and *SSS*-α-tocopherol), also found in fortified foods and supplements.

[e] As niacin equivalents (NE), 1 mg of niacin = 60 mg of tryptophan; 0–6 months = preformed niacin (not NE).

[f] As dietary folate equivalents (DFE), 1 DFE = 1 μg food folate = 0.6 μg of folic acid from fortified food or as a supplement consumed with food = 0.5 μg of a supplement taken on an empty stomach.

[g] Although AIs have been set for choline, there are few data to assess whether a dietary supply of choline is needed at all stages of the life cycle, and it may be that the choline requirement can be met by endogenous synthesis at some of these stages.

Dietary Reference Intakes (DRIs): Recommended Intakes for Individuals, Elements

Life Stage Group	Calcium (mg/d)	Chromium (µg/d)	Copper (µg/d)	Iron (mg/d)	Magnesium (mg/d)	Manganese (mg/d)	Molybdenum (µg/d)	Phosphorus (mg/d)	Selenium (µg/d)	Zinc (mg/d)	Potassium (g/d)
Children											
1–3 y	500*	11*	340	7	80	1.2*	17	460	20	3	3.0*
4–8 y	800*	15*	440	10	130	1.5*	22	500	30	5	3.8*
Males											
9–13 y	1,300*	25*	700	8	240	1.9*	34	1,250	40	8	4.5*
14–18 y	1,300*	35*	890	11	410	2.2*	43	1,250	55	11	4.7*
19–30 y	1,000*	35*	900	8	400	2.3*	45	700	55	11	4.7*
31–50 y	1,000*	35*	900	8	420	2.3*	45	700	55	11	4.7*
Females											
9–13 y	1,300*	21*	700	8	240	1.6*	34	1,250	40	8	4.5*
14–18 y	1,300*	24*	890	15	360	1.6*	43	1,250	55	9	4.7*
19–30 y	1,000*	25*	900	18	310	1.8*	45	700	55	8	4.7*
31–50 y	1,000*	25*	900	18	320	1.8*	45	700	55	8	4.7*

Recommended Dietary Allowances (RDAs) are in **bold type**, and Adequate Intakes (AIs) are in ordinary type followed by an asterisk(*).

Dietary Reference Intakes (DRIs): Tolerable Upper Intake Levels (UL^a), Vitamins

Life Stage Group	Vit.A (μg/d)^b	Vit.C (mg/d)	Vit.D (μg/d)	Vit.E (mg/d)^{c,d}	Vit.K	Thia-min	Ribo-flavin	Niacin (mg/d)^d	Vit.B$_6$ (mg/d)	Folate (μg/d)^d	Vit.B$_{12}$	Panto-thenic Acid	Biotin	Choline (g/d)
Children														
1–3 y	600	400	50	200	ND	ND	ND	10	30	300	ND	ND	ND	1.0
4–8 y	900	650	50	300	ND	ND	ND	15	40	400	ND	ND	ND	1.0
Males, Females														
9–13 y	1,700	1,200	50	600	ND	ND	ND	20	60	600	ND	ND	ND	2.0
14–18 y	2,800	1,800	50	800	ND	ND	ND	30	80	800	ND	ND	ND	3.0
19–>70 y	3,000	2,000	50	1,000	ND	ND	ND	35	100	1,000	ND	ND	ND	3.5

^{a} UL = The maximum level of daily nutrient intake that is likely to pose no risk of adverse effects. Unless otherwise specified, the UL represents total intake from food, water, and supplements. Due to lack of suitable data, ULs could not be established for vitamin K, thiamin, riboflavin, vitamin B$_{12}$, pantothenic acid, biotin, carotenoids. In the absence of ULs, extra caution may be warranted in consuming levels above recommended intakes.

^{b} As preformed vitamin A only.

^{c} As α-tocopherol; applies to any form of supplemental α-tocopherol.

^{d} The ULs for vitamin E, niacin, and folate apply to synthetic forms obtained from supplements, fortified foods, or a combination of the two.

ND = Not determinable due to lack of data of adverse effects in this age group and concern with regard to lack of ability to handle excess amounts. Source of intake should be from food only to prevent high levels of intake.

Dietary Reference Intakes (DRIs): Tolerable Upper Intake Levels (UL[a]), Elements

Life Stage Group	Calcium (g/d)	Chromium	Copper (µg/d)	Iron (mg/d)	Magnesium (mg/d)[b]	Manganese (mg/d)	Molybdenum (µg/d)	Phosphorus (g/d)	Potassium	Selenium (µg/d)	Zinc (mg/d)
Children											
1–3 y	2.5	ND	1,000	40	65	2	300	3	ND	90	7
4–8 y	2.5	ND	3,000	40	110	3	600	3	ND	150	12
Males, Females											
9–13 y	2.5	ND	5,000	40	350	6	1,100	4	ND	280	23
14–18 y	2.5	ND	8,000	45	350	9	1,700	4	ND	400	34
19–70 y	2.5	ND	10,000	45	350	11	2,000	4	ND	400	40

[a] UL = The maximum level of daily nutrient intake that is likely to pose no risk of adverse effects. Unless otherwise specified, the UL represents total intake from food, water, and supplements. Due to lack of suitable data, ULs could not be established for arsenic, chromium, silicon, potassium, and sulfate. In the absence of ULs, extra caution may be warranted in consuming levels above recommended intakes.

[b] The ULs for magnesium represent intake from a pharmacological agent only and do not include intake from food and water.

ND =Not determinable due to lack of data of adverse effects in this age group and concern with regard to lack of ability to handle excess amounts. Source of intake should be from food only to prevent high levels of intake.

The charts in Appendix 3 have been reprinted with permission from *Dietary Reference Intake: The Essential Guide to Nutrient Requirements* © 2006 by the National Academy of Sciences, courtesy of the National Academy Press, Washington, DC.

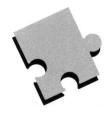

APPENDIX 4

IEP Nutrition Goals and Objectives

The following nutrition services are provided by schools participating in the School Nutrition Programs (National School Lunch and Breakfast) for children with disabilities.

INDIVIDUAL EDUCATION PROGRAM (IEP)

An IEP is a written plan for providing special education and related services to a child with a disability covered under the Individual Disabilities Education Act (IDEA). The IEP is the cornerstone of the child's education program and is designed to ensure that he receives the appropriate special education and related services to meet his educational needs. The IEP includes annual goals, short-term objectives, and an evaluation schedule.

An IEP offers an excellent opportunity to designate the required nutrition services to address your child's cognitive, educational, and nutritional needs. When a nutrition problem is identified for a child with a disability, a registered dietitian may be involved in the team meeting at the request of the parents or the school to participate in developing the child's IEP. Within an IEP, nutrition services may be specified as *special education* (specially designed instruction) or a *related service* (support services required to assist your child to benefit from his special education).

Here are some examples of ways to incorporate nutrition services into your child's IEP:

- His registered dietitian can consult with school food service staff to help meet your child's special nutritional needs.
- His registered dietitian can review and modify school menus to ensure they comply with your child's diet prescribed by his physician.

227

- Special education funds can be used to purchase special foods to accommodate your child's diet. This is especially helpful if your child is on the GFCF diet or needs other school meal modifications.

- School staff can give your child an afternoon snack two hours after lunch to help avoid a negative behavioral response to low blood sugar.

- School staff can develop and provide learning activities to teach your child about his dietary restrictions. This is especially helpful if your child is on the GFCF diet or has a life-threatening food allergy.

- An assigned school staff member can monitor your child at lunch to ensure compliance with diet restrictions. This is helpful if your child tends to take food from other children.

- The school nurse can measure your child's weight and height monthly, which is critical for children on stimulant medication that can affect their appetite and growth.

- A home economics teacher can teach your child about menu planning, grocery shopping, and food preparation skills. These are critical life skills for a high school student.

- A behavioral specialist can suggest a nonfood reward system/reinforcer to be used in place of food.

Disability Defined

The term *disability* under the Individuals with Disabilities Education Act (IDEA) recognizes thirteen disability categories, including autism, specific learning disabilities, and speech or language impairment. Attention deficit disorder or attention deficit hyperactivity disorder may fall under one of the thirteen categories.

SCHOOL MENU MODIFICATIONS

Substitutions or modifications to the school menu are allowed for children with a disability who are unable to eat a regular school meal. If you need to do this, your request to substitute or modify a school meal must be supported by a statement signed by a licensed physician. The medical statement must include the following information:

- Your child's disability.
- An explanation of why the disability restricts your child's diet.
- The major life activity affected by the disability. (Major life activity is defined as caring for one's self, doing manual tasks, walking, seeing, hearing, speaking, breathing, learning, and working).
- The food or foods to be omitted from your child's diet, and the food or choice of foods that must be substituted.

If your child has a disability that restricts his diet, he's entitled to modified school meals at no extra charge. Sources of funding to purchase special foods your child needs can include special education funds if the substitute food is specified in his IEP.

For more detailed information on this topic, as well as information on children *without* disabilities who have special dietary needs, read the USDA Food and Nutrition Services' "Accommodating Children with Special Dietary Needs in the School Nutrition Program," available at www.fns.usda.gov/cnd.

PHYSICIAN'S STATEMENT FOR CHILD WITH DISABILITY

Date: _____

Name of Child: _____ Date of Birth: _____

Child's disability: _____

_____

Describe why the disability restricts the child's diet:

_____

_____

_____

_____

Describe the major life activity affected by the child's disability:

_____

_____

_____

List food/foods to be omitted from the child's diet and the food or choice of foods that must be substituted:

_____

_____

_____

_____

_____   _____

Signature of Licensed Physician   Date

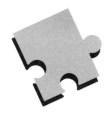

APPENDIX 5

Data Collection Forms

The purpose of a trial response is to help you determine which special diets and advanced nutritional supplements are beneficial for your child. The ultimate goal is to avoid keeping your child on an unnecessary restrictive diet or supplement.

These data collection forms were designed to provide you with a means to collect data and objectively determine if a special diet or advanced nutritional supplement is or is not beneficial for your child. A trial response is *not* necessary for a basic multivitamin and mineral or essential fatty acid supplement.

GENERAL GUIDELINES

- The final decision to perform a trial response on a special diet or nutritional supplement must be made by you. You should not feel pressured to try a nutrition intervention you're not comfortable with.

- Seek help from a registered dietitian when implementing any dietary changes, special diets, and advanced nutritional supplements.

- I advise you to seek the assistance from a supportive nutrition-oriented physician while implementing a trial response for medical supervision, monitoring, and joint-decision making purposes.

- Inform your child's therapists and teachers about the trial response and ask them to help by documenting their observations.

- You may also want to tell family members and other caregivers about the trial response to ensure the nutrition intervention is completely adhered to outside the home.

- Remember that you're actually performing a "mini experiment" on your child and you must remain objective, systematic, and observant and document all results.

INSTRUCTIONS

- Prior to the trial response, complete the following: Fill in the **baseline data** form.
- Describe in detail your child's current symptoms.
- Indicate the number of times per day, week, or month they occur. (This information is critical since it will be used to assess the effectiveness of the nutritional intervention at the completion of the trial response.)
- Request input from your child's therapists and teachers who work with your child on a regular basis. (Their information will be helpful regarding your child's current symptoms.)

TRIAL RESPONSE:

- With help from your child's registered dietitian, determine which nutrition intervention to try for your child.
- Don't initiate more than one *new* nutritional intervention at a time.
- Don't initiate a trial response if your child is starting a new medication for the first time.
- Determine the length of the trial response. The period of time for the trial response will vary based on the specific nutritional intervention. Here are some general guidelines for periods of time:

  Vitamin B₆: one month

  DMG: one month

  Gluten Free Casein Free Diet: three months

  Other nutrients: individualized—discuss with your child's registered dietitian.

  Elimination diet (food allergy/sensitivity/intolerance): individualized—discuss with your child's physician and/or registered dietitian.

- Initiate the new nutritional intervention for the trial response.
- Complete the **response data** form on a weekly basis to document your child's symptoms.

- Describe in detail your child's symptoms during the trial response.
- Gather input from your child's therapists and teachers regarding their documented observations of your child's symptoms during the trial response.

EVALUATION

- At the end of the trial response time period, evaluate the results of the nutritional intervention.
- Compare the response data to the baseline data.
- For each of your child's symptoms, determine if the nutritional intervention resulted in substantial improvement, some improvement, no change, or made things worse.
- Document your conclusions on the evaluation form.
- If you determine that the nutritional intervention made no difference or made your child's symptoms worse, stop the nutritional intervention. This particular nutrition intervention may *not* be beneficial for your child.
- If you determine the nutritional intervention resulted in substantial improvement and/or some improvement in one or more of your child's symptoms, continue the nutritional intervention. This particular nutrition intervention may be beneficial for your child.
- If you determine the nutritional intervention resulted in a combination of both positive and negative results, discuss the results with your child's physician and/or registered dietitian and decide if nutritional intervention should be continued.

BASELINE DATA FORM

Nutritional Intervention: _____

Date: _____

Symptom	*Describe in Detail Child's Symptoms*
Communication (verbal, speech, echolalia, conversation, eye contact)	
Social Interaction (interaction with others, social play, friendships)	
Behavior (self-injury, aggression, tantrums, resistant to change)	
Activities and Interest (stimming, pre-occupation with objects and/ or one interest)	
Sleep (falls asleep, stays asleep)	
Enuresis (bed wetting)	
Hyperactivity	
Focus and Attention	
Skin (eczema, hives, rashes)	
Ears (ear infections)	
Eyes (dark circles, red, itchy, watery)	
Respiratory (asthma, bronchitis, stuffy/ runny nose)	
Bowels (constipation, loose stools, diarrhea, gas, bloating)	
Feeding (limited variety of foods, refuse new foods)	

RESPONSE DATA FORM

Nutritional Intervention: _____

Dates: _____ **To** _____ **Week:** _____

Symptom	*Describe in Detail Child's Symptoms*
Communication (verbal, speech, echolalia, conversation, eye contact)	
Social Interaction (interaction with others, social play, friendships)	
Behavior (self-injury, aggression, tantrums, resistant to change)	
Activities & Interest (stimming, preoccupation with objects and/ or one interest)	
Sleep (falls asleep, stays asleep)	
Enuresis (bed wetting)	
Hyperactivity	
Focus and Attention	
Skin (eczema, hives, rashes)	
Ears (ear infections)	
Eyes (dark circles, red, itchy, watery)	
Respiratory (asthma, bronchitis, stuffy/runny nose)	
Bowels (constipation, loose stools, diarrhea, gas, bloating)	
Feeding (limited variety of foods, refuse new foods)	

EVALUATION FORM

Nutritional Intervention: _____

Date: _____

Symptom	Substantial Improvement	Improvement	No Change	Worsening
Communication (verbal, speech, echolalia, conversation, eye contact)				
Social Interaction (interaction with others, social play, friendships				
Behavior (self-injury, aggression, tantrums, resistant to change)				
Activities and Interest (stimming, preoccupation with objects and/or one interest)				
Sleep (falls asleep, stays asleep)				
Enuresis (bed wetting)				
Hyperactivity				
Focus and Attention				
Skin (eczema, hives, rashes)				
Ears (ear infections)				
Eyes (dark circles, red, itchy, watery)				
Respiratory (asthma, bronchitis, stuffy/runny nose				
Bowels (constipation, loose stools, diarrhea, gas, bloating)				
Feeding (limited variety of foods, refuse new foods)				

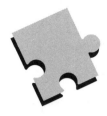

APPENDIX 6

Nutritional Detoxification Plan

Children live in a very toxic world today compared to a generation ago. There are more than eighty thousand chemicals in commercial use in the United States. More than 2.58 billion pounds of toxic chemicals are released into the air, water, and land by industrial facilities nationwide every year. More than 4.5 billion pounds of pesticide products are used each year as well. This means our children are exposed to a huge and ever-increasing number of toxic chemicals, which makes them more vulnerable to developmental, learning, and behavioral disabilities than previous generations. This is a major concern for parents, especially those in the autism community who are searching for safe, effective, and noninvasive ways to rid their children's bodies of toxins.

Below are a few basic nutritional steps you can take to naturally enhance your child's ability to detoxify. My plan will show you how to reduce his exposure to toxins, help him eat a more protective diet, and use additional helpful nutrients.

STEP 1: IDENTIFY AND ELIMINATE SOURCES OF TOXIN EXPOSURE

The most effective natural treatment is to identify the sources of toxins in your child's environment and eliminate his exposure to them. Following is a list of potential sources of toxins your child may come into contact with:

Home
- Age and condition of your home
- Recent renovation or home repairs
- Vinyl miniblinds manufactured in the 1990s
- Indoor and outdoor pesticides

- Sources of indoor heating, such as wood and gas stoves and fireplaces
- Radon (in homes with a basement)
- Indoor cigarette smoke
- Take-home exposure from parental occupations
- Parental hobbies, such as using an indoor firing range, arts and crafts, making stained glass
- Pressed-treated wood on deck and playground equipment
- Proximity of your home to a hazardous waste site
- Exposure to toxins at daycare, school, and play areas

Herbs, Nutritional Supplements, and Other Remedies
- Folk remedies contaminated with toxins such as lead, mercury, or arsenic
- Herbal products contaminated with toxins
- Herbal plants harvested from contaminated soils
- Multivitamin and mineral supplements contaminated with toxins

Drinking Water
- Unfiltered tap water can contain bacteria, viruses, parasites, natural toxins, inorganic and organic chemicals, disinfectants, and radon
- Private wells contaminated with pesticides

Food
- Food chemical additives, such as artificial colors, flavors, and preservatives
- Pesticide residue on fresh fruits and vegetables
- Bioaccumulative chemicals, such as dioxins and PCBs in fish
- Use of imported canned food products where the can is soldered with lead
- Food prepared in imported pottery or metal containers
- Excess consumption of fish contaminated with mercury

Behavioral Characteristics of Your Child
- Pica (eating nonfood items)
- Hand-to-mouth activity
- Doesn't wash his hands before meals and snacks

STEP 2: OPTIMIZE YOUR CHILD'S DIET

Nutrient deficiencies are associated with an increased absorption of toxins. It's critical that your child eat a wide variety of healthy foods from all the major food groups to ensure he's taking in enough amino acids, essential fatty acids, vitamins, and minerals. Mineral deficiencies especially put your child at risk for increased absorption of toxins.

For an adequate healthy diet, your child should:

- Eat a variety of foods that supply vitamins and minerals.
- Eat foods that are a good source of protein and critical minerals such as calcium, iron, and zinc.
- Identify and treat vitamin and mineral deficiencies in your child.
- Ask his pediatrician to do a laboratory test to identify iron deficiency anemia.
- Make sure he takes a daily multivitamin and mineral supplement that contains 100 to 300 percent of his RDA in all areas.

STEP 3: USE ADDITIONAL NUTRIENTS

Below is a list of additional nutrients that naturally support your child's detoxification function, which will help his body get rid of toxins more efficiently.

Alpha-Lipoic Acid. Dosage: Supplement intake ranges up to 600 mg per day in adults. Discuss proper dosage with your child's registered dietitian.

Glutathione. Glutathione in supplement form is not well-absorbed in the gastrointestinal tract, so it's not usually recommended as an oral supplement. Instead, I suggest you focus on increasing the amount of cysteine (precursor to glutathione) your child gets from dietary sources, such as beef, pork, chicken, turkey, eggs, milk, and whey protein.

N-acetylcysteine (NAC). Dosage: Supplement intake ranges up to 600 mg once to three times daily for adults. Discuss proper dosage with your child's registered dietitian.

Selenium. Dosage: Supplement intake ranges from at least 100 percent of your child's RDA, but should not exceed his UL. Turn to Appendix 3 to find your child's RDA and UL.

Trimethylglycine (TMG). Dosage: Supplement intakes typically range from 600–650 mg per day for adults. Discuss proper dosage with your child's registered dietitian.

Vitamin C. Dosage: Supplemental intake of 200 mg per day is enough to maximize plasma and lymphocyte levels; however, levels ranging from 500 to 2,000 mg are often suggested for adults. Do not exceed your child's UL for vitamin C without recommendation from his physician or registered dietitian. Turn to Appendix 3 for your child's UL.

Estimating Proper Dosage for Your Child

Often a therapeutic dosage for a particular nutrient, herb, or nutraceutical is suggested for an adult, but not a child. In this situation, your physician and/or registered dietitian will estimate your child's dosage. Here's the most common method used to estimate a child's dosage:

Adult Dosage ÷ 150 x Child's Weight = Child's Dosage

For example, the adult dosage suggested for alpha-lipoic acid is 600 mg. If a child weighs 35 pounds, how much is the estimated dosage for that child?

600mg ÷ 150 x 35 = 140 mg

Please keep in mind that this is only an estimate, and your child's physician and/or registered dietitian will make adjustments based on his unique needs.

For additional information on environmental toxins, sources of exposure, body systems affected, effects on development and cognitive function, diagnostic testing, and treatment, I suggest the following resources:

Etzel, R. and S. Balk (eds). *Pediatric Environmental Health* (2nd ed.). Elk Grove Village, IL: American Academy of Pediatrics 2003.

In Harm's Way: Toxic Threats to Child Development. A Report by Greater Boston Physicians for Social Responsibility Prepared for a Joint Project with Clean Water Fund. May 2000. Available at www.igc.org/psr.

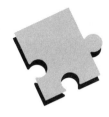

APPENDIX 7

Laboratory Tests

WHAT LAB TESTS DOES MY CHILD NEED?

Many laboratory tests marketed directly to the autism community are very controversial and may not be reliable or helpful in choosing the appropriate nutritional interventions for your child. These tests are usually not covered by health insurance and may cost a family thousands of dollars out of pocket. I prefer to utilize standardized lab tests that are available through any commercial lab and reimbursed by insurance companies with a physician's order.

Below is a list of basic lab tests to assist you and your child's registered dietitian in individualizing his nutrition plan.

- Complete Blood Count (CBC)
- Comprehensive Metabolic Panel (CMP)
- Blood Lead
- Thyroid Function (T3, T4, TSH)
- IgE RAST (basic foods)
- IgE RAST (airborne allergens)
- Carnitine (free, total, and acylcarnitine)
- Specific Vitamins and Minerals (these will be individualized based on your child's medications, suspected nutrient deficiencies, clinical history, and other factors)

Your physical may recommend additional lab tests to assess your child's immune function, identify gastrointestinal disorders, and address any other health concerns. More detailed information on lab tests is available at www.nlm.nih.gov/medlineplus/laboratorytests.

GLOSSARY

Acetylcholinesterase. An enzyme that helps break down the neurotransmitter acetylcholine, producing choline.

Adrenaline. Also called epinephrine, it's a "fight or flight" hormone produced by the adrenal glands. It elevates heart and respiration rates, elevates blood sugar, and suppresses the immune system.

Allergen. A substance that the body recognizes as foreign and provokes an immune response, which causes the allergy reaction.

Alpha-tocopherol. The most active form of vitamin E.

Amino acids. The building blocks of proteins. There are twenty standard amino acids, with eight considered essential.

Anal fissure. Crack or tear in the anus that can cause bleeding and pain after a bowel movement.

Anaphylaxis. A severe, life-threatening allergic response that may be characterized by symptoms such as lowered blood pressure, wheezing, vomiting or diarrhea, and swelling and hives.

Antifungals. Herbs or drugs used to treat fungal infections.

Aspartame. A sugar substitute that's about two hundred times sweeter than table sugar. Also known as Equal and NutraSweet.

Aspartic acid. A nonessential amino acid found in animal sources and a few vegetable sources. It's used to produce the artificial sweetener aspartame.

Aspiration. Inhalation of food or liquid into the trachea (windpipe) and lungs.

Autistic enterocolitis. The controversial term used to describe a number of common gastrointestinal symptoms that seem to be distinctive to autism.

Avenin. The prolamin (group of plant proteins high in the amino acids proline and glutamine) found in oats.

Betaine. Another name for trimethylglycine (TMG), a water-soluble substance related to choline involved in the S-Adenosyl-L-Methionine (SAMe) pathway.

Biopsy. The removal of cells or tissues for examination under a microscope.

Blood-brain barrier (BBB). A structure of tight junctions in the central nervous system that restricts the passage of various chemicals and bacteria between the bloodstream and neural tissue.

Butylated hydroxyanisole (BHA) and butylated hydroxytoluene (BHT). Fat-soluble organic compounds used as an antioxidant food additive. It's also used in cosmetics, pharmaceutical drugs, jet fuels, rubber, petroleum products, and embalming fluid.

Candida albicans. A form of yeast that lives in the gastrointestinal tract. Under normal conditions it has no harmful effect; however, overgrowth results in candidiasis.

Carbohydrate. The main source of energy for the body that's composed of starches and sugars. Carbohydrates are found predominantly in breads, cereals, pastas, rice, beans, potatoes, fruits, and vegetables.

Caries. A term for tooth decay or cavities.

Carotenoids. A collection of plant pigments that are found in yellow, orange, red, and dark green fruits and vegetables.

Casein. A protein found in milk and milk products.

Casomorphine. A peptide, or short chain of amino acids, derived from the incomplete digestion of casein.

Central nervous system. The part of the nervous system consisting of the brain and spinal cord. Along with the peripheral nervous system, it plays a major role in the control of behavior.

Coal tar. A by-product of coal when it's carbonized to make fuel or gasified to make coal gas. When combined with phenols and other compounds it's used to make artificial colors.

Colitis. Inflammation of the colon.

Colonoscopy. A test that uses a long, flexible tube passed through the anus to take pictures inside the large intestines (colon) and distal part of the small intestines. It has the ability to cut off polyps and tissue samples.

Complementary protein. A plant protein source that is incomplete on its own, but when combined with another incomplete protein, provides the balance of amino acids necessary to form a complete protein.

Complete protein. A protein that contains all the essential amino acids in amounts required to meet the dietary needs of humans. Sources include meat, fish, poultry, eggs, milk, and soy.

Complex carbohydrates. Known as "starchy" foods, complex carbs are good sources of energy and nutrients, such as whole grain breads and cereals, starchy vegetables, and legumes.

Cross contamination. The term used to describe when a safe food (food that doesn't contain any allergens) comes in contact with an allergen during its production, preparation, cooking, storage, or serving.

Cytokines. A protein involved in cellular communication. It's secreted by immune cells to activate more immune cells to respond to an allergen.

Dehydration. When not enough water is taken in or the loss of too much body fluid through urine, sweat, diarrhea or vomit.

Delta 6 desaturase. Enzyme involved in the lipid metabolic pathway that converts essential fatty acids into long-chain polyunsaturated fatty acids. For example, linoleic acid converts to gamma linolenic acid (GLA) and alpha linolenic acid (ALA) converts to EPA and DHA.

Dietary Reference Intake (DRI). A system of nutrition recommendations that was introduced in 1997 in order to broaden the existing guidelines known as Recommended Dietary Allowances (RDA). It includes four nutrient-based values: the EAR, RDA, AI, and the UL.

Digestive enzymes. Enzymes secreted by glands in the mouth, stomach, and small intestines that break down food. Proteases and peptidases split protein into amino acids, lipases split fat into fatty acids, and carbohydrases split carbohydrate into sugars.

Dihydroxyphenyl isatin. A chemical found in prunes known to stimulate bowel movements.

Docosahexaenoic acid (DHA). The most abundant fatty acid found in the brain and retina, this omega-3 fatty acid is essential to the growth and functional development of the brain.

Dopamine. A neurotransmitter that has numerous important functions in the brain involving mood, attention, learning, cognition, motor activity, and motivation and reward.

Duodenitis. Inflammation of the duodenum (first part of small intestines) where most of digestion takes place.

Dysbiosis. The imbalance of microorganisms (yeast, helpful bacteria, harmful bacteria) in the gastrointestinal tract.

Eicosanoids. A family of powerful, hormone-like compounds produced in the body from 20-carbon essential fatty acids. Eicosanoids derived from omega-6 fatty acids are pro-inflammatory.

Encopresis. Occurs when a person resists having a bowel movement, causing impacted stool to collect in the colon and rectum. The large intestine get stretched to the point where liquid stool leaks around the impacted stool and passes through the anus into the child's underwear.

Eosinophilic colitis (EC). An allergic inflammatory condition of the colon.

Eosinophilic esophagitis (EE). An allergic inflammatory condition of the esophagus.

Eosinophilic gastroenteritis (EG). An allergic inflammatory condition of the stomach and small intestines.

Eosinophilic gastrointestinal disorders (EGID). A complex group of disorders characterized by having excessive amounts of eosinophils in the digestive tract. Symptoms vary depending on the area affected, and include swallowing difficulty, heartburn, poor appetite, diarrhea, bloating, chest and abdominal pain, and difficulty sleeping.

Eosinophils. A type of white blood cell that can increase in response to an allergy and other infections. It controls mechanics associated with allergies.

EPIPEN. A device used to inject epinephrine to treat anaphylactic shock.

Erythropoiesis. The process of producing red blood cells that transport oxygen to the brain and throughout the body.

Esophagitis. An inflammation of the lining of the esophagus, usually caused by a backflow of acid from the stomach.

Essential fatty acids. These are the fats the body cannot make and therefore must be part of the diet. There are two groups, omega-3 (alpha-linoleic acid) and omega-6 fatty acids (linoleic acid).

Excitotoxin. A substance in excess amounts that can cause overactivity of the excitatory neurotransmitters in the brain, resulting in injury or death to these neurons. Glutamic acid is classified as an excitotoxin.

Fat. An essential nutrient that provides energy, energy storage, insulation to the body, transports fat-soluble vitamins, and is critical for brain function.

Food allergen. A food that the body recognizes as foreign and provokes an immune response which causes an allergic reaction.

Food protein-induced enterocolitis. A gastrointestinal condition resulting in inflammation of the small and large intestines caused by a non-IgE mediated food allergy.

Gastroenteritis. Inflammation of the stomach and small intestines that may be caused by a virus, bacteria, parasites, or an adverse reaction to a food. Symptoms include acute diarrhea, nausea and vomiting, abdominal pain and cramping, loss of appetite, and bloody stools.

Gastritis. An inflammation of the stomach lining caused by viruses, bacteria, fungus, use of alcohol, and prolonged use of certain drugs. Symptoms include abdominal pain, nausea and vomiting, bloating, and loss of appetite.

Gastric-emptying study. A procedure that measures the speed at which food empties from the stomach and enters the small intestines.

"Generally recognized as safe" (GRAS). An FDA designation that a chemical or substance added to food is considered safe for the general public and poses no significant health hazard.

Gliadomorphine. A peptide, or short chain of amino acids, derived from the incomplete digestion of gluten.

Glossitis. An inflammation of the tongue.

Glucose oxidation. The breakdown of glucose to produce ATP, which transports energy within cells.

Glutathione. A tripeptide made within the body from the amino acids cysteine, glutamate, and glycine. It functions as a cofactor for the glutathione S-transferase enzymes involved in the detoxification of chemical toxins.

Glycemic index (GI). The ranking of carbohydrate-containing foods based on the food's effect on blood sugar levels. The higher the GI score, the faster the release of glucose into the bloodstream and the more rapid a rise in the blood sugar level.

High-fructose corn syrup (HFCS). Regular corn syrup that has been processed to increase its fructose content, then mixed with pure corn syrup. It's sweeter than table sugar (sucrose).

Hippotherapy. A form of medical therapy that uses the movement of a horse to provide sensory input as a means to treat movement dysfunction. Specially trained occupational, physical, or speech therapists use hippotherapy to improve a child's balance, posture, and mobility.

Histamine. A naturally occurring substance present in cells throughout the body that is released by the immune system after exposure to an allergen and causes an allergic reaction.

Homocysteine. A chemical compound similar to the amino acid cysteine that the body converts to methionine and then to SAMe.

Hydrogen breath test. A test that measures the amount of hydrogen and methane gases in the breath and helps diagnose lactose intolerance, fructose malabsorption, and overgrowth of intestinal bacteria.

Hydrogenation. The process whereby hydrogen is added to a liquid vegetable oil and changes the oil to a soft or solid state. It produces a more malleable fat that's solid at room temperature but melts upon baking.

Hyperglycemia. A condition commonly known as "high blood sugar" in which there is an excess amount of glucose in the blood.

Hypertonia. A condition marked by an abnormal increase in the tightness of muscle tone and a reduced ability of a muscle to stretch.

Hypoglycemia. A condition commonly known as "low blood sugar" in which there is a low amount of glucose in the blood.

Hypotonia. A condition of abnormally low muscle tone in skeletal muscles.

Hypervitaminosis A. A term that refers to the adverse effects of excessive vitamin A intake, specifically as preformed vitamin A in supplement form.

IgE mediated food allergy. Triggered by a food allergen, the immune system responds by releasing immunoglobulin E (IgE) antibodies to bind with the food allergen and cause an allergic reaction.

Incomplete protein. A protein that's lacking one or more of the essential amino acids. Sources include grains, beans, peas, nuts, seeds, and a few vegetables.

Insoluble fiber. A type of fiber that absorbs water as it passes through the intestinal tract, softening stool, increasing stool bulk, and promoting bowel movements. It's mainly found in whole grain products, bran, nuts, seeds, vegetables, and skin of fruits.

Insulin. A hormone released by the pancreas that causes glucose to move from the blood into the cells in the body, where it can be used to produce energy.

Interleukins. A group of cytokines produced naturally in the body to regulate inflammation and immune responses.

Intravenous immune globulin (IVIG). A treatment in which IgG immunoglobulins (antibodies from plasma of blood donors) are administrated intravenously (directly into a vein). It's used to treat immune deficiencies, inflammatory, and autoimmune diseases.

Lactose intolerance. The inability to digest milk and milk products due to a deficiency of the enzyme lactase, which breaks down milk sugar (lactose). The undigested lactose passes from the small intestines into the colon, causing abdominal symptoms.

Leaky gut syndrome. A condition in which there is increased intestinal permeability of the intestinal wall, making it more permeable than normal. This allows large, intact protein molecules to pass into the bloodstream.

Leavening. A substance used in doughs and batters that causes a foaming action intended to lighten and soften the finished baked product. The most common leaveners are yeast, baking powder, and baking soda.

Lower esophageal sphincter. The muscle lying at the end of the esophagus and opening of the stomach that relaxes to let food enter the stomach, then closes to prevent stomach acid from entering the esophagus.

Lymphonodular hyperplasia (LNH). Lymphoid tissue mass found in the small intestines or colon associated with food allergies resulting in abdominal pain.

Megacolon. A condition in which the colon enlarges and dilates. Feces can consolidate in the colon resulting in chronic constipation.

Minerals. Naturally occurring inorganic elements that come from the soil and water and are essential for maintaining and sustaining our body. Various plants and/or animals absorb minerals, and we need to eat these plants and/or animals to obtain these minerals.

Modified barium swallow study. X-ray procedure also known as a *video fluoroscopic swallow study (VFSS)* that's used to determine whether an individual is able to swallow safely without aspirating food or liquid into his lungs.

Monosodium glutamate (MSG). An additive used to commercially enhance the flavor of processed and pre-packaged foods.

Motor dysfunction. An abnormality of brain function that directs purposeful muscle movement activity.

Mucosa. Also called the mucous membrane, it's the moist tissue that lines body cavities exposed to the external environment (such as the nostrils, lips, ears, and anus) and internal organs (such as the lungs). The thick fluid secreted by mucous membranes is called mucus.

Myelin sheath. The fatty layer of insulation surrounding the axons of neurons increasing the speed at which electrical impulses can travel from neuron to neuron.

Natural killer cells. Also known as NK cells, they're a type of white blood cell that attacks infected body cells and releases lethal chemicals, killing abnormal cells before they multiple and grow.

Neurons. Cells in the central and peripheral nervous systems that process and transmit information through chemical signals.

Neurotransmitter. A chemical that relays signals between a neuron and another cell. Stored in vesicles in the presynaptic terminals, neurotransmitters are released by an electrical stimulation into the synapse and then bind with receptors on the postsynaptic terminal of another cell. Examples of neurotransmitters are acetylcholine, norepinephrine, dopamine, serotonin, melatonin, glutamate, gamma aminobutyric acid, aspartate, glycine, histamine, and purines.

Non-IgE mediated food allergy. Unlike an IgE mediated food allergy reaction, the immune system does not release IgE antibodies. Instead it responds directly to a food protein by releasing certain chemicals. This leads to inflammation that causes a variety of milder reactions throughout the body, but primarily in the gastrointestinal tract.

Obsessive-compulsive disorder (OCD). An anxiety disorder characterized by recurrent, repetitive thoughts (obsessions), repetitive behaviors (compulsions), or a combination of both. A person with OCD recognizes that his obsessions and compulsions are unreasonable or excessive.

Oligomeric proanthocyanidins (OPC). A class of flavonoids that act as an antioxidant with numerous reported health benefits. Found in grape seed, grape skin, red wine, pine bark, apples, cranberries, green and black tea, and cocoa.

Opiate peptides. Peptides with opiate-like analgesic actions and characteristics similar to morphine. They're believed to play a role in causing behavioral disturbances.

Oral immunoglobulin (OIG). An encapsulated form of intravenous immunoglobulin (IVIG) for oral use. OIG is considered a biomedical treatment and used by complementary and alternative physicians to treat immune system disorders.

Oral tolerance test. A test where the individual consumes a designated amount of lactose, then his serum glucose level is measured at certain time intervals. A diagnosis of lactose intolerance is confirmed according to the level of glucose above baseline.

Organochlorides. These are chlorinated hydrocarbons that belong to a class of chemicals that can cause significant toxicity to humans. They are commonly used in many pesticides.

Osmotic diarrhea. Occurs when too much water is drawn into the bowels. It can result from maldigestion of food, undigested lactose, and too much magnesium or vitamin C in supplement form.

Partially hydrogenated. A term that refers to a liquid oil that's been hydrogenated (hydrogen atoms are added to the oil), which makes it more saturated. Hydrogenation results in a more solid product, such as tub margarine and shortening, which is more appropriate for baking.

Peripheral nervous system. The nerves connecting the central nervous system to the limbs and organs.

pH probe study. Also called pH monitoring, it's a procedure used to determine if stomach acid is coming up into the esophagus.

Phenol sulfotransferase (PST). A key enzyme in the liver responsible for processing and eliminating phenols and other toxic substances from the body.

Phenylalanine. An essential amino acid found in protein foods. The body converts naturally occurring L-phenylalanine to tyrosine, which is essential for making proteins, neurotransmitters, and thyroid hormones. The synthetic forms D and DL-phenylala-nine may cause adverse reactions in the body.

Prealbumin. One of several plasma proteins. It can be measured in a laboratory test to as-sess protein status.

Prebiotic. A food ingredient that promotes the growth of helpful bacteria in the gas-trointestinal tract.

Preformed vitamin A. The type of vitamin A found in animal sources that occurs in a form ready to be used by the body.

Primary carnitine deficiency. A genetic disorder where a child's carnitine transporters don't work properly and prevent the body from properly using fats for energy. It mani-fests by five years of age.

Probiotic. Live microorganisms that are similar to the beneficial "good bacteria" found in the gut. They can help improve the microflora balance in the gastrointestinal tract by in-hibiting the presence of other, harmful microorganisms.

Prostaglandins. Hormone-like compounds derived from essential fatty acids that are in-volved in constriction or dilation of smooth muscle, aggregation or disaggregation of platelets, control of cell growth, and regulation of inflammation.

Protein. Large organic compounds made of amino acids required for the structure, func-tion, and regulation of the body's cells, tissues, and organs. They participate in every process within cells.

Reactive hypoglycemia. An abnormal spike in blood glucose level due to eating a food or meal high in carbohydrate which triggers the pancreas to release an excess amount of in-sulin to lower the blood glucose level. This in turn causes the blood glucose level to drop rapidly (reactive hypoglycemia), triggering the release of adrenaline and other hormones to raise the blood glucose level once again.

Retinol binding protein. A family of protein that has a diverse number of functions. They are carriers of protein that bind retinol (preformed vitamin A) and can be measured in a laboratory test to assess visceral protein mass related to nutritional health.

Saccharin. Also known as Sweet'N Low, this sugar substitute is about three-hundred to five-hundred times sweeter than table sugar.

S-Adenosyl-L-Methionine (SAMe). A coenzyme involved in methyl group transfer. SAMe may have a positive effect on mood, emotional well-being, and depression. It also plays a role in detoxification by increasing glutathione levels in the liver.

Salicylates. Chemicals that occur naturally in many plants.

Selenosis. Poisoning by selenium caused by consuming an excess amount of selenium over a short or long-term time period.

Sensory integration dysfunction (SID). A neurological disorder causing difficulties with processing information from the five classic senses (vision, auditory, touch, olfaction, and taste), the sense of movement (vestibular system), and/or the positional sense (proprioception). Also known as sensory processing disorder (SPD).

Sensory neuropathy. A condition of the peripheral nerves that causes numbness, tingling, and burning sensations commonly in the hands, arms, feet, and legs.

Serotonin. A neurotransmitter in the central nervous system that regulates mood, aggression, anger, sleep, and appetite.

Serum albumin. A major protein found in the blood that transports drugs and other substances, and is important for keeping fluid from leaking out of blood vessels into the tissues. It can be measured in a laboratory test to assess protein status.

Serum ferritin test. A laboratory test used to measure the amount of iron in the blood and provides an indirect measure of the body's iron stores. Ferritin is a protein inside cells that store iron in the body for later use.

Simple carbohydrate. A major type of carbohydrate that's broken down quickly by the body to be used as energy. They occur naturally in fruits, milk, and milk products and are also found in processed foods like table sugar, candy, and soft drinks.

Soluble fiber. Soluble fiber resists digestion and absorption in the small intestines and promotes the proliferation of helpful bacteria in the large intestine, lowers cholesterol levels, and stabilizes blood sugar levels. It's found mainly in beans, peas, soybeans, psyllium seed husk, oats, barley, fruits, prune juice, and root vegetables.

Sucralose. Also known as Splenda, this sugar substitute is about six hundred times sweeter than table sugar.

Sucrose. A disaccharide of glucose and fructose. More commonly known as white sugar or table sugar.

Total iron binding capacity (TIBC) test. A laboratory test that measures the extent to which iron binding sites can be saturated, indicating if there is iron deficiency or iron overload. If your iron level is low, the TIBC will be elevated.

Transfer factors. Immune messengers found in white blood cells, colostrum, and eggs. These messengers transfer immunity against pathogens to the immune cells of the recipient.

Transferrin. A blood plasma protein that binds with iron to transport iron in the blood. It can be measured in a laboratory test to assess protein status.

Ubiquinones. Water-soluble substances that function as coenzymes and are involved in electron transport and energy production in the mitochondria.

Upper GI endoscopy. A procedure where a thin, flexible viewing instrument (endoscope) is inserted through the mouth, into the esophagus, stomach, and upper part of the small intestines (duodenum). This allows a physician to look for abnormalities and take tissue samples.

Upper GI X-ray. A test used to help identify problems in the upper gastrointestinal tract, including the esophagus, stomach, and upper part of the small intestines (duodenum). A special X-ray (fluoroscopy) is taken after swallowing barium, making it possible to see internal organs in motion.

Videofluoroscopic swallow study (VFSS). An X-ray procedure that's used to determine whether an individual is able to swallow safely without aspirating food or liquid into his lungs. Also known as a modified barium swallow study.

Vitamins. Organic components in food that are needed in very small amounts to perform diverse functions, such as regulation of cell and tissue growth, processing and eliminating toxins from the body, maintaining a healthy gastrointestinal tract, supporting immune function, and forming blood. Some vitamins also function as hormones, antioxidants, coenzymes, and precursors for enzymes.

RESOURCES

Nutrition Therapy

Elizabeth Strickland, M.S., R.D., L.D.
ASD Nutrition Seminars & Consulting
P.O. Box 1495
Canyon Lake, TX 78133
Phone: (830) 237-2886
Fax: (866) 855-8301
Email: ASDpuzzle@aol.com

Web site: www.ASDpuzzle.com

Elizabeth provides the following services:
   Speaking engagements
   Seminars for professionals
      (offering CEU)
   Workshops for parent groups
   Nutrition Assessment/Consultation
      (nationwide via telephone)

Organizations

These organizations provide detailed
information and helpful resources for
managing autism:

Autism Research Institute
4182 Adams Avenue
San Diego, CA 92116
Phone: (619) 281-7165
Web site: www.autism.com

Autism Society of America (ASA)
7910 Woodmont Avenue, Suite 300
Bethesda, MD 20814-3067
Phone: (800) 328-8476
Web site: www.autism-society.org

Cure Autism Now Foundation
5455 Wilshire Blvd.
Suite 2250
Los Angeles, CA 90036
Phone: (323) 549-0500
Email: contactus@autismspeaks.org
Web site: www.cureautismnow.org

Families for Early Autism Treatment
   (FEAT)
P.O. Box 255722
Sacramento, CA 95865-5722
Phone: (916) 491-1033
Email: feat@feat.org
Web site: www.feat.org

National Autism Association
1330 W. Schatz Road
Nixa, MO 65714
Phone: (877) 622-2884
Email: naa@nationalautism.org
Web site: www.nationalautism
   association.org

National Institute of Child Health and
 Human Development (NICHD)
National Institutes of Health, Autism
 Research at NICHD
P.O. Box 3006
Rockville, MD 20847
Phone: (800) 370-2943
Email: NICHDinformationresourcecenter
 @mail.nih.gov
Web site: www.nichd.nih.gov/autism

Talk About Curing Autism
3070 Bristol Street, Suite 340
Costa Mesa, CA 92626
Phone: (949) 640-4401
Web site: www.tacanow.com

Nutritional Supplements

Virtually all of the nutritional supplements
discussed in this book can be purchased
through these two sources:

Kirkman
6400 SW Rosewood Street
Lake Oswego, OR 97035
Phone: (800) 245-8282
Fax: (503) 682-0838
Email: sales@kirkmanlabs.com
Web site: www.kirkmangroup.com

Village Green Apothecary
5415 W. Cedar Lane
Bethesda, MD 20814
Phone: (800) 869-9159 (store)
Phone: (301) 530-1112 (compounding)
Fax: (301) 493-4671
Email: info@myvillagegreen.com
Web site: www.the-apothecary.com

Professional Referrals

These organizations can help you find
qualified therapists to work with your child:

American Dietetic Association (ADA)
216 West Jackson Blvd.
Chicago, Illinois 60606
Web site: www.eatright.org

American Speech Language and Hearing
 Association (ASHA)
10801 Rockville Pike
Rockville, Maryland 20852
Phone: (800) 638-8255
Web site: www.asha.org

American Occupational Therapist
 Association
4720 Montgomery Lane
P.O. Box 31220
Bethesda, MD 20824-1220
Phone: (800) 377-8555
Web site: www.aota.org

Behavior Analysis Certification Board
Metro Building
Suite 102
1705 Metropolitan Blvd.
Tallahassee, Florida 32308-3796
Web site: www.bacb.com

Food Allergy Resources

American Academy of Allergy, Asthma, and
 Immunology
555 East Wells Street, Suite 1100
Milwaukee, Wisconsin 53202-3823
Phone: (414) 272-6071
Email: info@aaaai.org
Web site: www.aaaai.org

Asthma and Allergy Foundation of America
1233 20th Street NW, Suite 402
Washington, D.C. 20036
Phone: (800) 727-8462
Email: info@aafa.org
Web site: www.aafa.org

Food Allergy and Anaphylaxis Network
11781 Lee Jackson Hwy, Suite 160
Fairfax, Virginia 22033-3309
Phone: (800) 929-4040
Email: faan@foodallergy.org
Web site: www.foodallergy.org

Product Sources for Gluten Free Casein Free Diet
Allergy Grocer
91 Western Maryland Parkway, Unit 7
Hagerstown, MD 21740
Phone: (800) 891-0083
Email: info@allergygrocer.com
Web site: www.allergygrocer.com

Bob's Red Mill Natural Foods
5000 SE International Way
Milwaukie, OR 97222
Phone: (800) 349-2173
Web site: www.bobredmil.com

Dietary Specialties
10 Leslie Court
Whippany, NJ 07981
Phone: (888) 640-2800
Email: info@dietspec.com
Web site: www.dietspec.com

Ener-G Foods
5960 First Avenue South
P.O. Box 84487
Seattle, WA 98124
Phone: (800) 331-5222
Web site: www.ener-g.com

Enjoy Life Foods
3810 River Road
Schiller Park, IL 60176
Phone: (847) 260-0300
Web site: www.enjoylifefoods.com

Laurel's Sweet Treats
8174 SW Durham Road
Tigard, OR 97224
Phone: (866) 225-3432
Email: sales@glutenfreemixes.com
Web site: www.glutenfreemixes.com

Pamela's Products
200 Clara Avenue
Ukiah, CA 95842
Phone: (707) 462-6605
Email: info@pamelasproducts.com
Web site: www.pamelasproducts.com

Vance's Foods
P.O. Box 627
Gilmer, TX 75644
Phone: (800) 497-4834
Email: info@vancesfoods.com
Web site: www.vancesfoods.com

Helpful Web Sites

The following Web sites offer reliable information on many of the topics discussed in this book, such as herbal medicine, CAM, and special elimination diets:

American Botanical Council,
    www.herbalgram.org

Andrew Weil, M.D., www.drweil.com

Consumer Lab, www.consumerlab.com

Feingold Association, www.feingold.org

MEDLINEplus, www.medlineplus.com

National Center for Complementary
    and Alternative Medicine,
    www.nccam.nih.gov

NSF International, www.nsf.org

Nutrition in Complementary Care,
    www.complementarynutrition.org

Office of Dietary Supplements,
    National Institute of Health (NIH),
    www.ods.od.nih.gov

The GFCF Diet Support Group,
    www.gfcfdiet.com

US Pharmacopeia (USP), www.usp.org

Recommended Reading

Fraker, Cheri, M. Fishbein, S. Cox, and L. Walbert. *Food Chaining: The Proven 6-Step Plan to Stop Picky Eating, Solve Feeding Problems, and Expand Your Child's Diet* (Boston: Da Capo Press, 2007).

Seminars for Professionals and Parents

Feeding Problems

Kay Toomey, Ph.D.
Toomey & Associates, Inc.
1780 South Bellaire Street, Suite 515
Denver, CO 80012
Phone: (303) 759-5316
Fax: (303) 759-5320

Special Education and Advocacy

Peter Wright, Esq.
P.O. Box 1008
Deltaville, VA 23043
Web site: www.wrightslaw.com

Nutrition and Autism

Elizabeth Strickland, M.S., R.D., L.D.
P.O. Box 1495
Canyon Lake, TX 78133
Phone: (830) 237-2886
Email: ASDpuzzle@aol.com
Web site: www.ASDpuzzle.com

BIBLIOGRAPHY

Introduction

Alberti, A., et al. "Sulphation deficit in 'low-functioning' autistic children—a pilot study." *Biological Psychiatry* 46 (1999):420–424.

Burger, S., et al. "Testing the effects of nutrient deficiencies on behavioral performance." *American Journal of Clinical Nutrition* S57 (1993):295S–302S.

Conners, K. and A. Blouin. "Nutrition effects on behavior of children." *Journal of Psychiatric Research* 117, no. 21 (1982/83):193–201.

Curtis, L. and K. Patel. "Nutritional and environmental approaches to preventing and treating autism and attention deficit hyperactivity disorder (ADHD): A review." *Journal of Alternative and Complementary Medicine* (2008 Jan 16).

Harrington, J.W., et al. "Parental perceptions and use of complementary and alternative medicine practices for children with autistic spectrum disorders in private practice." *Journal of Developmental and Behavioral Pediatrics* 27, (2006):S156–161.

Jackson, K. "Nutrition and autism: Are they linked?" *Today's Dietitian* 7 (2005):31.

Knivsberg, A., et al. "A randomized, controlled study of dietary intervention in autistic syndromes." *Nutritional Neuroscience* 5, no. 4 (2002):251–261.

———. "Reports on dietary intervention in autistic disorders." *Nutritional Neuroscience* 4, no. 1 (2001):25–37.

Lanphear, B., et al. "Cognitive deficits associated with blood lead concentrations <10 microg/dL. U.S. children and adolescents." *Public Health Reports* 115 (2000):521–529.

Latif, A., P. Heinz, and R. Cook. "Iron deficiency in autism and Asperger syndrome." *Autism* 6, no. 1 (Mar 2002):103–114.

Levy, S., et al. "Use of complementary and alternative medicine among children recently diagnosed with autistic spectrum disorder." *Journal of Developmental and Behavioral Pediatrics* 24 (2003):418–423.

McFadden, S. "Phenotypic variation in xenobiotic metabolism and adverse environmental response: Focus on sulfur-dependent detoxification pathways." *Toxicology* VIII (1996):43–65.

Page, T. "Metabolic approaches to the treatment of autism spectrum disorders." *Journal of Autism and Developmental Disorders* 30, no. 5 (Oct 2000):463–469.

Patel, K. and L. Curtis. "A comprehensive approach to treating autism and attention-deficit hyperactivity disorder: A prepilot study." *Journal of Alternative and Complementary Medicine* 13, no. 10 (Dec 2007):1091–1098.

Peregrin, T. "Registered dietitians' insights in treating autistic children." *Journal of the American Dietetic Association* 107, no. 5 (May 2007):727–730.

Potts, M. and B. Bellows. "Autism and diet." *Journal of Epidemiology and Community Health* 60, no. 5 (May 2006):375.

Schnoll, R., D. Burshteyn, and J. Cea-Aravena. "Nutrition in the treatment of attention-deficit hyperactivity disorder: A neglected but important aspect." *Applied Psychophysiology and Biofeedback* 28, no. 1 (Mar 2003):63–75.

Wong, H., and R. Smith. "Patterns of complementary and alternative medical therapy use in children diagnosed with autism spectrum disorders." *Developmental Disorders* 36 (2006):901–909.

Wurtman, R. "Ways that foods can affect the brain." *Nutrition Review* 5, no. S (1986):2.
———. "Behavioral effects of nutrients." *Lancet* 1 (1983):1145.

Zeisel, S. "Dietary influences on neurotransmission." *Advances in Pediatrics* 33 (1986): 23–47.

Step 1

Agricultural Marketing Service, U.S. Department of Agriculture. USDA Organic. Available at http://www.ams.usda.gov.

Alavanja, M., J. Hoppin, and F. Kamel. "Health effects of chronic pesticide exposure: Cancer and neurotoxicity." *Annual Review of Public Health* 25 (2004):155–197.

Bateman, B., et al. "The effects of a double blind, placebo controlled, artificial food colorings and benzoate preservative challenge on hyperactivity in a general population sample of preschool children." *Archives of Disease in Childhood* 89, no. 6 (Jun 2004):506–511.

Behar, D., et al. "Sugar challenge testing with children considered behaviorally sugar reactive." *Nutrition and Behavior* 1 (1984):277–288.

Bellinger, D. "Children's cognitive health: The influence of environmental chemical exposures." *Alternative Therapies in Health and Medicine* 13, no. 3 (Mar–Apr 2007):S140–144.

Boris, M. and F. Mandel. "Foods and additives are common causes of the attention deficit hyperactive disorder in children." *Annals of Allergy, Asthma and Immunology* 72, no. 5 (May 1994):462–468.

Carter, C., et al. "Effects of a few food diets in attention deficit disorder." *Archives of Disease in Childhood* 69, no. 5 (Nov 1993):564–568.

Chensheng, L. "Organic diets significantly lower children's dietary exposure to organophosphorus pesticides." *Environmental Health Perspectives* 114 (2006):260–263.

Cruz, N. and S. Bahna. "Do food or additives cause behavior disorders?" *Pediatrics Annals* 35, no. 10 (Oct 2006):744–745, 748–754.

Eskenazi, B., A. Bradman, and R. Castorina. "Exposures of children to organophosphate pesticides and their potential adverse health effects." *Environmental Health Perspective* 107 (1999):409–419.

Ferguson, H., et al. "Food dyes and impairment of performance in hyperactive children." *Science* 211, no. 4480 (Jan 1981):410–411.

Fuglsang, G., et al. "Adverse reactions to food additives in children with atopic symptoms." *Allergy* 49, no. 1 (Jan 1994):31–37.

———. "Prevalence of intolerance to food additives among Danish school children." *Pediatric Allergy and Immunology* 4, no. 3 (Aug 1993):123–129.

Goldman, J., et al. "Behavioral effects of sucrose on preschool children." *Journal of Abnormal Child Psychology* 14 (1986):565–578.

Hunter, J.E. "Dietary levels of trans fatty acids basis for health concerns and industry efforts to limit use." *Nutrition Research* 25 (2005):499–513.

Jacobson, M., et al. "Diet, ADHD & Behavior: A Quarter-Century Review." Center for Science in the Public Interest 1999 September. 1875 Connecticut Ave. NW #300, Washington, DC 2009.

Jones, et al. "Enhanced adrenomedullary response and increased susceptibility to neuroglycopenia mechanisms underlying adverse effects of sugar ingestion in healthy children." *Journal of Pediatrics* 126, no. 2 (Feb. 1995):171–177.

Kamel, F. and J. Hoppen. "Association of pesticide exposure with neurological dysfunction and disease." *Environmental Health Perspectives* 112 (2004):950–958.

Kamel, F. "Neurobehavioral performance and work experience in Florida farmworkers." *Environmental Health Perspectives* 111 (2003):1765–1772.

Kaplan B, et al. "Dietary replacement in preschool-aged hyperactive boys." *Pediatrics* 83 (1989):7–17.

Madsen, C. "Prevalence of food additive intolerance." *Human and Experimental Toxicology* 13, no. 6 (Jun 1994):393–399.

Mahfouz, M. "Effect of dietary trans fatty acids on the delta 5, delta 6, and delta 9 desaturases of rat liver microsomes in vivo." *Acta biologica et medica germanica* 40, no. 12 (1981):1699–1705.

Mattes, J. and R. Gittelman. "Effects of artificial food colorings in children with hyperactive symptoms: A critical review and results of a controlled study." *Archives of General Psychiatry* 38, no. 6 (Jun 1981):714–718.

McCann, D., et al. "Food additives and hyperactive behaviour in 3-year-old and 8/9-year-old children in the community: A randomized, double-blinded, placebo-controlled trial." *Lancet* 3, no. 9598 (Nov 2007):1560–1567.

McLoughlin, J. and M. Nall. "Teacher opinion of the role of food allergy on school behavior and achievement." *Annals of Allergy* 61 (1988):89–91.

Meldrum, B. "Amino acids as dietary excitotoxins: A contribution to understanding neurodegenerative disorders. Brain research." *Brain research review* 18, no. 3 (1993):293–314.

Milich, R., et al. "The effects of sugar ingestion on the classroom and playgroup behavior of attention deficit disordered boys." *Journal of Consulting & Clinical Psychology* 54 (1986):1–5.

Olney, J. "Excitotoxins in foods." *Neurobehavioral toxicology and teratology* 15, no. 3 (1994):535–544.

O'Reilly, B. and R. Waring. "Enzyme and sulphur oxidation deficiencies in autistic children with known food/chemical intolerances." *Journal of Orthomolecular Medicine* 8 (1993):198–200.

Printz, R., et al. "Sugar consumption and hyperactivity in young children." *Journal of Consulting & Clinical Psychology* 48 (1980):760–769.

Rohlman, D., et al. "Neurobehavioral performance in preschool children from agricultural and non-agricultural communities in Oregon and North Carolina." *Neurotoxicology* 26, no. 4 (Aug 2005):589–598.

Rowe, K., et al. "Synthetic food coloring and behavior; A dose response effect in a double-blind, placebo-controlled, repeated-measures study." *Journal of Pediatrics* 125 (1994):691–698.

Rowe, K.S. "Synthetic food colorings and 'hyperactivity': A double-blind crossover study." *Australian Paediatrics Journal* 24, no. 2 (Apr 1988):143–147.

Salamy, J., et al. "Physiological changes in hyperactive children following the ingestion of food additives." *International Journal of Neuroscience* 16, no. 3–4 (May 1982):241–246.

Schab, D. and N. Trinh. "Do artificial food colors promote hyperactivity in children with hyperactive syndromes? A meta-analysis of double-blind placebo-controlled trials." *Journal of Developmental and Behavioral Pediatrics* 25, no. 6 (Dec 2004):423–434.

Schnoll, R., D. Burshteyn, and J. Cea-Aravena. "Nutrition in the treatment of attention-deficit hyperactivity disorder: A neglected but important aspect." *Applied Psychophysiology Biofeedback* 28, no.1 (Mar 2003):63–75.

Schoenthaler, S., W. Doraz, and J. Wakefield. "The impact of a low food additive and sucrose diet on academic performance in 803 New York City public schools." *International Journal of Biosocial and Medical Research* 8, no. 2 (1986)185–195.

Swanson, J., et al. "Food dyes impair performance of hyperactive children on a laboratory learning test." *Science* 207, no. 4438 (Mar 28 1980):1485–1487.

Veien, N., et al. "Oral challenge with food additives." *Contact Dermatitis* 17, no. 2 (Aug 1987):100–103.

Weiss, B., et al. "Behavioral responses to artificial food colors." *Science* 207, no. 4438 (Mar 28 1980):1487–1489.

Wilson, N., et al. "A double-blind assessment of additive intolerance in children using a 12-day challenge period at home." *Clinical and Experimental Allergy* 19, no. 3 (May 1989):267–272.

Wolraich, M., et al. "Effects of diets high in sucrose or aspartame on the behavior and cognitive performance of children." *New England Journal of Medicine* 3, no. 5 (Feb 1994):301–307.

Zeisel, S. "Dietary influences on neurotransmission." *Advances in Pediatrics* 33 (1986): 23–47.

Step 2

American Academy of Pediatrics. "A summary of conference recommendations on dietary fiber in childhood." Conference on Dietary Fiber in Childhood, New York, May 24, 1994. *Pediatrics* 96 (1995):1023–1028.

ADA Pocket Guide to Pediatric Nutrition Assessment. First Edition. Beth Leonberg, MS, MA, RD, LDN. Published by American Dietetic Association, January 2008.

Arnold, G., et al. "Plasma amino acids profiles in children with autism: Potential risk of nutritional deficiencies." *Journal of Autism and Developmental Disorders* 33, no. 4 (Aug 2003):449–454.

B vitamins, calcium, and iron. National Institutes of Health. Office of Dietary Supplements. Available at http://ods.od.nih.gov.

Carbohydrate and Dietary Fiber. Kleinman, RE, et al. *Pediatric Nutrition Handbook* (5th ed.) Elk Grove Village, IL. American Academy of Pediatrics, 2004, 247–259.

Fat. Kleinman, R.E., et al. *Pediatric Nutrition Handbook* (5th ed.) Elk Grove Village, IL. American Academy of Pediatrics, 2004, 261–278.

Food and Nutrition Board, Institute of Medicine, National Academies. Dietary Reference Intakes for Energy, Carbohydrate, Fiber, Fat, Fatty Acids, Cholesterol, Protein, and Amino Acids (2002).

Froster-Iskenius, U., et al. "Folic acid treatment in males and females with fragile X syndrome." *American Journal Medical Genetics* 23 (1986):273–289.

Konofal, E., et al. "Iron supplementation may help children with ADHD." *Archives of Pediatrics and Adolescent Medicine* 158 (2004):1113–1115.

Leonberg, B.L. *ADA Pocket Guide to Pediatric Nutrition Assessment.* Elk Grove Village, IL. American Dietetic Association, 2008.

Meldrum, B. "Amino acids as dietary excitotoxins; A contribution to understanding neurodegenerative disorders. Brain research." *Brain research reviews* 18, no. 3 (1993): 293–314.

Munoz, K.A., et al. "Food intakes of U.S. children and adolescents compared with recommendations." *Pediatrics* 100, no. 3 (1997):323–329.

Nutrient Data Laboratory, United States Department of Agriculture. USDA National Nutrient Database for Standard Reference. Available at http://www.nal.usda.gov/fnic/foodcomp.

Protein. Kleinman, R.E., et al. *Pediatric Nutrition Handbook* (5th ed.) Elk Grove Village, IL. American Academy of Pediatrics, 2004, 229–240.

Richardson, A.J., et al. "Fatty acid metabolism in neurodevelopmental disorder: A new perspective on associations between attention deficit/hyperactivity disorder, dyslexia, dyspraxia, and the autistic spectrum." *Prostaglandins, Leukotrines, and Essential Fatty Acids* 63 (2000):1–9.

Reynolds, K. "The prevalence of nitrate contamination in the United States." *Water Conditioning and Purification* 44, no. 1 (2002).

U.S. Environmental Protection Agency, Office of Water. A Review of Contaminant Occurrence in Public Water Systems. Washington, DC. U.S. Environmental Protection Agency; 1999. EPA Publication 816-R-99-006.

Williams, C., M. Bollella, and E. Wynder. "A new recommendation for dietary fiber in childhood." *Pediatrics* 96 (1995):985–988.

Wurtman, R. "Effects of dietary amino acids, carbohydrates, and choline on neurotransmitter synthesis." *Mt. Sinai Journal of Medicine* 55 (1988):75.

Step 3

Adams, J. and C. Holloway. "Pilot study of a moderate dose multivitamin/mineral supplement for children with autistic spectrum disorder." *Journal of Alternative and Complementary Medicine* 10, no. 6 (Dec 2004):1033–1039.

Benton, D., et al. "The impact of long-term vitamin supplementation on cognitive function." *Psychopharmacology* 117 (1995):298–305.

Hediger, M.L. "Thin bones seen in boys with autism and autism spectrum disorder." Published online in *Journal of Autism and Developmental Disorders.* January 2008.

National Institutes of Health. Office of Dietary Supplements. Available at http://www.dietary-supplements.info.nih.gov.

Nutrient Data Laboratory, United States Department of Agriculture. USDA National Nutrient Database for Standard Reference. Available at http://www.nal.usda.gov/fnic/foodcomp.

United States National Library of Medicine. Dietary Supplements Labels Database. Available at http://www.dietarysupplements.nlm.nih.gov/gov/dietary/index.

Step 4

Antalis, C., et al. "Omega-3 fatty acid status in attention-deficit/hyperactivity disorder." *Prostaglandins Leukotrines and Essentials Fatty Acids* 75, no. 4–5 (Oct–Nov 2006):299–308.

Aman, M., E. Mithell, and S. Turbott. "The effects of essential fatty acid supplementation by Efamol in hyperactive children." *Journal of Abnormal Child Psychology* 15, no. 1 (Mar 1987):75–90.

Amminger, G., et al. "Omega-3 fatty acids supplementation in children with autism: A double-blind randomized, placebo-controlled pilot study." *Biological Psychiatry* 61, no.4 (2007):551–553.

Arnold, L., et al. "Does Zinc moderate essential fatty acids and amphetamine treatment of attention-deficit/hyperactivity disorder?" *Journal of Childhood Adolescent Psychopharmacology* 10, no. 2 (Summer 2000):111–117.

———. "Potential link between dietary intake of fatty acids and behavior: Pilot exploration of serum lipids in Attention-Deficit Hyperactivity Disorder." *Journal of Child and Adolescent Psychopharmacology* 4 (1994):171–182.

———. "Gamma-linolenic acid for attention-deficit hyperactivity disorder: Placebo-controlled comparison to D-amphetamine." *Biological Psychiatry* 25, no. 2 (Jan 15 1989): 222–228.

Bekaroglu, M., et al. "Relationships between serum free fatty acids and zinc and attention deficit hyperactivity disorder: A research note." *Journal of Child Psychology and Psychiatry* 37, no. 2 (Feb 1996):225–227.

Bell, J., et al. "Essential fatty acids and phospholipase A2 in autistic spectrum disorders." *Prostaglandins, Leukotrienes and Essential Fatty Acids* 71, no. 4 (Oct 2004):201–204.

Burgess, J., L. Stevens, W. Zhang, and L. Peck. "Long-chain polyunsaturated fatty acids in children with attention-deficit hyperactivity." *American Journal of Clinical Nutrition* 71, no. 1 (Jan 2000):327S-330S.

Center for Food Safety and Applied Nutrition, U.S. Food and Drug Administration. An important message for pregnant women and women of childbearing age, who may become pregnant, about the risks of mercury in fish. Washington, DC. U.S. Food and Drug Administration; 2001. Available at http://vm.cfsan.fda.gov.

Cormier, E. and J. Elder. "Diet and child behavior problems: Fact or fiction?" *Pediatric Nursing* 33, no. 2 (Mar–Apr 2007):138–143.

Food Nutrition Board, Institute of Medicine, National Academies. AI for ALA. Available at www.iom.edu.

Glen, A., et al. "A red cell membrane abnormality in a subgroup of schizophrenic patients: Evidence for two diseases." *Schizophrenic Research* 12 (1994):53–61.

Haag, M. "Essential fatty acids and the brain." *Canadian Journal of Psychiatry* 48, no.3 (Apr 2003):195–203.

Hallahan, B. and M. Garland. "Essential fatty acids and their role in the treatment of impulsivity disorder." *Prostaglandins Leukotrienes and Essential Fatty Acids* 71, no. 4 (Oct 2004):211–216.

Hibbeln, J. "Fish consumption and major depression." *Lancet* 351 (1998):1213

Hunter, J.E. "Dietary levels of trans fatty acids basis for health concerns and industry efforts to limit use." *Nutrition Research* 25 (2005):499–513.

Johnson, S. and E. Hollander. "Evidence that eicosapentaenoic acid is effective in treating autism." *Journal of Clinical Psychiatry* 64, no. 7 (2003):848–849.

Joshi, K., et al. "Supplementation with flax oil and vitamin C improves the outcome of Attention Deficit Hyperactivity Disorder (ADHD)." *Prostaglandins, Leukotrienes and Essential Fatty Acids* 74, no. 1 (Jan 2006):17–21.

Kidd, P. "Attention deficit/hyperactivity disorder (ADHD) in children: Rationale for its integrative management." *Alternative Medicine Review* 5, no. 5 (Oct 2000):402–428.

Mahfouz, M. "Effect of dietary trans fatty acids on the delta 5, delta 6, and delta 9 desaturases of rat liver microsomes in vivo." *Acta biologica et medica germanica* 40, no. 12 (1981):1699–1705.

Melanson, S., et al. "Fish oil supplements may be safer than eating fish." *Archives of Pathology and Laboratory Medicine* 129 (2005):74-77.

Mithell, E., M. Aman, S. Turbot, and M. Manku. "Clinical characteristics and serum essential fatty acid levels in hyperactive children." *Clinical Pediatrics* 26, no. 8 (Aug 1987):406–411.

National Institutes of Health. Available at www.hhs.gov.

Nemets, et al. "Addition of omega-3 fatty acid to maintenance medication treatment for recurrent unipolar depressive disorder." *American Journal of Psychiatry* 159 (2002):477–479.

Richardson, A. "Omega-3 fatty acids in ADHD and related neurodevelopmental disorders." *International Review of Psychiatry* 18, no. 2 (2006):144-172.

Richardson, A. and P. Montgomery. "The Oxford-Durham Study: A randomized, controlled trial of dietary supplementation with fatty acids in children with developmental coordination disorder." *Pediatrics* 115, no. 5 (2005):1360–1366.

Richardson, A., et al. "The potential role of fatty acids in attention-deficit/hyperactivity disorder." *Prostaglandins, Leukotrienes and Essential Fatty Acids* 63, no. 1–2 (Jul–Aug 2000):79–87.

Richardson, A. and M. Ross. "Fatty acid metabolism in neurodevelopmental disorder: A new perspective on association between attention-deficit/hyperactivity disorder, dyslexia, dyspraxia, and the autistic spectrum." *Prostaglandins, Leukotrienes and Essential Fatty Acids* 63 (2000):1–9.

Simopoulos, A. "The importance of the ratio of omega-6/omega-3 essential fatty acids." *Biomedicine & Pharmacotherapy* 56 (2002):365–379.

Sinn, N. "Physical fatty acid deficiency signs in children with ADHD symptoms." *Prostaglandins, Leukotrienes, and Essential Fatty Acids* 77, no. 2 (Aug 2007):109–115.

Sinn, N. and J. Bryan. "Effect of supplementation with polyunsaturated fatty acids and micronutrients on learning and behavior problems associated with child ADHD." *Journal of Developmental and Behavioral Pediatrics* 28, no. 2 (Apr 2007):82–91.

Sliwinski, S., et al. "Polyunsaturated fatty acids: Do they have a role in the pathophysiology of autism?" *Neuroendocrinology Letters* 27, no. 4 (Aug 2006):465–471.

Stevens, L., et al. "Omega-3 fatty acids in boys with behavior, learning, and health problems." *Physiology and Behavior* 59 (1996):915–920.

————. "Essential fatty acid metabolism in boys with Attention-Deficit Hyperactivity Disorder." *American Journal of Clinical Nutrition* 62, no. 4 (Oct 1995):761–768.

Stoll, A., et al. "Omega 3 fatty acids in bipolar disorder." *Archives of General Psychiatry* 56 (1999):407–412.

Stordy, J. "Dark adaptation, motor skills, docosahexaenoic acid, and dyslexia." *American Journal of Clinical Nutrition* 71, no. 1 Suppl (Jan 2000):323S–326S.

————. "Benefit of docosahexaenoic acid supplements to dark adaptation." *Lancet* 346 (1995):8971.

Stradomska, T., et al. "Very long-chain fatty acids in Rett syndrome." *European Journal of Pediatrics* 158 (1999):226–229.

Tsalamanio, E., A. Yanni, and C. Koutsari. "Omega-3 fatty acids: Role in the prevention and treatment of psychiatric disorders." *Current Psychiatry Review* 2, no. 2 (2006):215–234.

U.S. Environmental Protection Agency on fish Advisories. Available at www:epa.gov/fishadvisories.

Vancassel, et al. "Plasma fatty acid levels in autistic children." *Prostaglandins, Leukotrienes and Essential Fatty Acids* 65, no. 1 (Jul 2001):1–7.

Wainwright, P. "Dietary essential fatty acids and brain function: A developmental perspective on mechanisms." *Proceedings of the Nutrition Society* 61 (2002):61–69.

Weber, W. and S. Newmark. "Complementary and alternative medical therapies for attention-deficit/hyperactivity disorder and autism." *Pediatric Clinics of North America* 54, no. 6 (Dec 2007):983–1006.

Willatts, P., et al. "The role of long-chain polyunsaturated fatty acids in infant cognitive development." *Prostaglandins, Leukotrienes and Essential Fatty Acids* 63 (2000): 95–100.

Young, G., J. Conquer, and R. Thomas. "Effect of randomized supplementation with high dose olive, flax, or fish oil on serum phospholipids fatty acid levels in adults with attention deficit hyperactivity disorder." *Reproduction Nutrition Development* 45, no. 5 (Sep–Oct 2005):549–558.

Young, G. and J. Conquer. "Omega-3 fatty acids and neuropsychiatric disorders." *Reproduction Nutrition Development* 45, no. 1 (2005):1–28.

Step 5

Ahearn, W., et al. "An assessment of food acceptance in children with autism or pervasive developmental disorder—not otherwise specified." *Journal of Autism and Developmental Disorders* 31, no. 5 (Oct 2001):505–511.

Efron, L. "Use of extinction and reinforcement to increase food consumption and reduce expulsion." *Journal of Applied Behavior Analysis* 30 (1997):581–583.

Field, D., M. Garland, and K. Williams. "Correlates of specific childhood feeding problems." *Journal of Paediatric and Child Health* 39, no. 4 (May–Jun 2003):299–304.

Fraker, C., M. Fishbein, S. Cox, and L. Walbert. *Food Chaining: The Proven 6-Step Plan to Stop Picky Eating, Solve Feeding Problems, and Expand Your Child's Diet.* New York. Marlowe & Company 2007.

Luiselli, J. "Oral feeding treatment of children with chronic food refusal and multiple developmental disabilities." *American Journal on Mental Retardation* 98, no. 5 (1994):646–655.

Ogata, B. "Autism, nutrition, and the picky eater." *Developmental Issues* 18, no. 4 (2000):1–5.

Pronsky, Z. *Food Medication Interactions* (15th Ed). Birchrunville, PA. Food Medication Interactions 2008.

Raiten, D. and T. Massaro. "Perspectives on the nutritional ecology of autistic children." *Journal of Autism and Developmental Disorders* 16, no. 2 (Jun 1986):133–143.

Riordan, M., et al. "Behavioral assessment and treatment of chronic food refusal in handicapped children." *Journal of Applied Behavior Analysis* 17 (1984):327–341.

Schreck, K. and K. Williams. "Food preferences and factors influencing food selectivity for children with autism spectrum disorders." *Research in Developmental Disabilities* 27, no. 4 (Jul–Aug 2006):353–363.

Schreck, K., K. Williams, and A. Smith. "A comparison of eating behaviors between children with and without autism." *Journal of Autism and Developmental Disorders* 34, no. 4 (Aug 2004):433–438.

Schwarz, S., et al. "Diagnosis and treatment of feeding disorders in children with developmental disabilities." *Pediatrics* 108, no. 3 (Sep 2001):671–676.

Seabert, H., E. Eastwood, and A. Harris. "A multiprofessional children's feeding clinic." *Journal of Family Health Care* 15, no. 3 (2005):72–74.

Werle, M., et al. "Treating chronic food refusal in young children: Home-based parent training." *Journal of Applied Behavior Analysis* 26 (1993):421–433.

Williams, P., N. Dalrymple, and J. Neal. "Eating habits of children with autism." *Pediatric Nursing* 26, no. 3 (May–Jun 2000):259–264.

Step 6

Afzal, N., S. Murch, K. Thirrupathy, L. Berger, A. Fagbemi, and R. Heuschkel. "Constipation with acquired megarectum in children with autism." *Pediatrics* 112, no. 4 (Oct 2003):939–942.

Ashwood, P. and A. Wakefield. "Immune activation of peripheral blood and mucosal CD3+ lymphocyte cytokine profiles in children with autism and gastrointestinal symptoms." *Journal of Neuroimmunology* 173, no. 1–2 (Apr 2006):126–134.

Ashwood, P., et al. "Spontaneous mucosal lymphocyte cytokine profiles in children with autism and gastrointestinal symptoms: Mucosal immune activation and reduced counter regulatory interleukin-10." *Journal of Clinical Immunology* 24, no. 6 (Nov 2004): 664–673.

————. "Intestinal lymphocyte populations in children with regressive autism: Evidence for extensive mucosal immunopathology." *Journal of Clinical Immunology* 23, no. 6 (Nov 2003):504–517.

Balzola, F., et al. "Panenteric IBD-like disease in a patient with regressive autism shown for the first time by the wireless capsule enteroscopy: Another piece in the jigsaw of this gut-brain syndrome?" *American Journal of Gastroenterology* 100, no. 4 (Apr 2005):979–981.

Black, C., J. Kaye, and H. Jick. "Relation of childhood gastrointestinal disorder to autism: Nested case-control study using data from the UK General Practice Research Database." *British Medical Journal* 325 (2002):419–421.

Boorom, K. "Is this recently characterized gastrointestinal pathogen responsible for rising rates of inflammatory bowel disease (IBD) and IBD associated autism in Europe and the United States in the 1990s?" *Medical Hypotheses* 69, no. 3 (2007):652–659.

DeFelice, M., et al. "Intestinal cytokines in children with pervasive developmental disorders." *American Journal of Gastroenterology* 98, no. 8 (Aug 2003):1777–1782.

D'Eufemia, P., et al. "Abnormal intestinal permeability in children with autism." *Acta Paediatricaica* 85, no. 9 (Sep 1996):1076–1079.

Dhillon, A. "Autistic enterocolitis: Is it a histopathological entity?" *Histopathology* 50, no. 6 (Feb 2007):794.

Erickson, C., et al. "Gastrointestinal factors in autistic disorder. a critical review." *Journal of Autism and Developmental Disorders* 35, no. 6 (Dec 2005):713–727.

Fernell, E., U. Fagerberg, and P. Hellstrom. "No evidence for a clear link between active intestinal inflammation and autism based on analyses of faecal calprotectin and rectal nitric oxide." *Acta Paediatricaics* 96, no. 7 (Jul 2007):1076–1079.

Finegold, S., et al. "Gastrointestinal microflora studies in late-onset autism." *Clinical Infectious Diseases* 1, no. 35 (Sep 2002):S6–16.

Fombonne, E. "Inflammatory bowel disease and autism." *Lancet* 351, no. 9107 (Mar 28 1998):955.

Furlano, R., et al. "Colonic CD8 and gamma delta T-cell infiltration with epithelial damage in children with autism." *Journal of Pediatrics* 138, no. 3 (Mar 2001):366–372.

Garvey, J. "Diet in autism and associated disorders." *Journal of Family Health Care* 12, no. 2 (2002):34–38.

Goldbert, E. "The link between gastroenterology and autism." *Gastroenterology Nursing* 27, no.1 (Jan–Feb 2004):16–19.

Horvath, K. and J. Perman. "Autism and gastrointestinal symptoms." *Current Gastroenterology Report.* 4, no. 3 (Jun 2002):251–258.

————. "Autistic disorder and gastrointestinal disease." *Current Opinion in Pediatrics* 14, no. 5 (Oct 2002):583–587.

————. "Autism and gastrointestinal symptoms." *Current Gastroenterology Reports* 4, no. 3 (Jun 2002):251–258.

Horvath, K., et al. "Gastrointestinal abnormalities in children with autistic disorder." *Journal of Pediatrics* 135, no. 5 (Nov 1999):559–563.

Jass, J. "The intestinal lesion of autistic spectrum disorder." *European Journal of Gastroenterology & Hepatology* 17, no. 8 (Aug 2005):821–822.

Jyonouchi, H., et al. "Dysregulated innate immune responses in young children with autism spectrum disorders: Their relationship to gastrointestinal symptoms and dietary intervention." *Neuropsychobiology* 51, no. 2 (2005):77–85.

Kemperman, R., et al. "Normal intestinal permeability at elevated platelet serotonin levels in a subgroup of children with pervasive developmental disorder in Curacao (The Netherlands Antilles)." *Journal of Autism and Developmental Disorders* 38, no. 2 (Feb 2008):401–406.

Kuddo, T. and K. Nelson. "How common are gastrointestinal disorder in children with autism?" *Current Opinion in Pediatrics* 15, no. 3 (Jun 2003):339–343.

Levy, S., et al. "Relationship of dietary intake to gastrointestinal symptoms in children with autistic spectrum disorders." *Biological Psychiatry* 61, no. 4 (Feb 2007):492–497.

Levy, S. and S. Hyman. "Novel treatments for autistic spectrum disorders." *Mental Retardation and Developmental Disabilities Research Reviews* 11, no. 2 (2005):131–142.

Lightdale. J., B. Siegel, and M. Heyman. "Gastrointestinal symptoms in autistic children." *Clinical Perspectives in Gastroenterology* 1 (2001):56–58.

Linday, L. "*Saccharomyces boulardii*: Potential adjunctive treatment for children with autism and diarrhea." *Journal of Child Neurology* 16, no. 5 (May 2001):387.

Liu, Z., N. Li, and J. Neu. "Tight junctions, leaky intestines, and pediatric diseases." *Acta Paediatrica* 94, no. 4 (Apr 2005):386–393.

MacDonald, T. and P. Domizio. "Autistic enterocolitis: Is it a histopathological entity?" *Histopathology* 50, no. 3 (Feb 2007):371–379; discussion 380-384.

MacDonald, T. "The significance of ileocolonic lymphoid nodular hyperplasia in children with autistic spectrum disorder." *European Journal of Gastroenterology & Hepatology* 18, no. 5 (May 2006):569–571.

McGinnis, W. "Mercury and autistic gut disease." *Environmental Health Perspectives* 109, no. 7 (Jul 2001):A303–304.

Melmed, R., et al. "Metabolic markers and gastrointestinal symptoms in children with autism and related disorders (abstract)." *Journal of Pediatric Gastroenterology and Nutrition* 31, no. 12 (2003):S31.

Molloy, C. and P. Manning-Courtney. "Prevalence of chronic gastrointestinal symptoms in children with autism and autistic spectrum disorders." *Autism* 7, no. 2 (Jun 2003):165–171.

Murch, S. "Separating inflammation from speculation in autism." *Lancet* 362, no. 9394 (Nov 2003):1498–1499.

Natural Health Products Directorate of Canada. Available at: www.hc-sc.gc.ca.

Niehus, R. and C. Lord. "Early medical history of children with autism spectrum disorders." *Journal of Developmental and Behavioral Pediatrics* 27, no.2 (Apr 2006):S120–127.

Quigley, E. and D. Hurley. "Autism and the gastrointestinal tract." *American Journal of Gastroenterology* 95, no. 9 (Sep 2000):2154–2156.

Robertson, M., et al. "Intestinal permeability and glucagon-like peptide-2 in children with autism: A controlled pilot study." *Journal of Autism and Developmental Disorders* (Feb 29 2008) Epub ahead of print.

Senior, K. "Possible autoimmune enteropathy found in autistic children." *Lancet* 359, no. 9318 (May 11 2002):1674.

Taylor, B., et al. "Measles, mumps, and rubella vaccination and bowel problems or developmental regression in children with autism. population-based study." *British Medical Journal* 324, (2002):393–396.

Torrente, F., et al. "Focal-enhanced gastritis in regressive autism with features distinct from Crohn's and Helicobacter pylori gastritis." *American Journal of Gastroenterology* 99, no. 4 (Apr 2004):598–605.

———. "Small intestinal enteropathy with epithelial IgG and complement deposition in children with regressive autism." *Molecular Psychiatry* 7, no. 4 (2002):375–382, 334.

Uhlmann, V., et al. "Potential viral pathogenic mechanism for new variant inflammatory bowel disease." *Molecular Pathology* 55, no. 2 (Apr 2002):84–90.

Valicenti-McDermott, M., et al. "Frequency of gastrointestinal symptoms in children with autistic spectrum disorders and association with family history of autoimmune disease." *Journal of Developmental and Behavioral Pediatrics* 27, no. 2 (2006):S128–136.

Van, H., S. Jones, and M. Giacomantonio. "Rectal prolapse in autistic children." *Journal of Pediatric Surgery* 39, no. 4 (Apr 2004):643–644.

Wakefield, A., et al. "The significance of ileo-colonic lymphoid nodular hyperplasia in children with autistic spectrum disorder." *European Journal of Gastroenterology & Hepatology* 17, no. 8 (Aug 2005):827–836.

———. "Review article: The concept of entero-colonic encephalopathy, autism, and opioid receptor ligands." *Alimentary Pharmacology & Therapeutics* 16, no. 4 (Apr 2002):663–674.

———. "Enterocolitis in children with developmental disorders." *American Journal of Gastroenterology* 95, no. 9 (Sep 2000):2285–2295.

———. "Ileal-lymphoid-nodular hyperplasia, non-specific colitis, and pervasive developmental disorder in children." *Lancet* 351 (2000):637–641.

———. "Ileal-lymphoid-nodular hyperplasia, non-specific colitis, and pervasive developmental disorder in children." *Lancet* 351, no. 9103 (Feb 28 1998):637–641.

Wakefield, A. "Enterocolitis, autism, and measles virus." *Molecular Psychiatry* 7, no. 2 (2002):S44–46.

———. "The gut-brain axis in childhood developmental disorders." *Journal of Pediatric Gastroenterology and Nutrition* 34, no. 1 (May–Jun 2002):S14–17.

White, J. "Intestinal pathophysiology in autism." *Experimental Biology and Medicine* 228, no. 6 (Jun 2003):639–649.

Step 7

Anderson, J. " Mechanisms in adverse reactions to food: The brain." *Allergy* 50, no. 20 (1995):78–81.

Atkinson, W., et al. *Gut* 53 (Oct 2004):1459–1464.

Boris, M., et al. "Foods and additives are common causes of Attention Deficit Hyperactive Disorder in Children." *Annals of Allergy, Asthma and Immunology* 72 (1994):462–468.

Carter, C., et al. "Effects of a few food diet in Attention Deficit Disorder." *Archives of Disease in Childhood* 69 (1993):564–568.

Christison, G.W. and K. Ivany. "Elimination diets in autism spectrum disorders: Any wheat amidst the chaff?" *Journal of Developmental and Behavioral Pediatrics* 27, no. 2 (2006):S162–171.

Dolovich, J. "Attention deficit disorder and food intolerance." *Canadian Medical Association Journal* 147, no. 12 (Dec 15 1992):1755.

Egger, J., A. Stolla, and L. McEwen. "Controlled trial of hyposensitization in children with food-induced hyperkinetic syndrome." *Lancet* 339, no. 8802 (May 9 1992):1150–1153.

Egger, J., et al. "Controlled trail of oligoantigenic treatment in the hyperkinetic syndrome." *Lancet* 1, no. 8428 (Mar 1985):540–545.

Franklin, A. "Hyposensitization for food-induced hyperkinetic syndrome." *Lancet* 341, no. 8842 (Feb 13 1993):437.

Hadjivassiliou, M., et al. "Wheat protein can trigger severe headaches." *Neurology* 56 (2001):385–388.

Jacobson, M., et al. "Diet, ADHD & Behavior: A Quarter-Century Review." Center for Science in the Public Interest, Sep 1999. 1875 Connecticut Ave. NW #300, Washington, DC 20009.

Jyonouchi, H., et al. "Dysregulated innate immune responses in young children with autism spectrum disorders: Their relationship to gastrointestinal symptoms and dietary intervention." *Neuropsychobiology* 51, no. 2 (2005):77–85.

Kaplan, B., et al. "Dietary replacement in preschool-aged hyperactive boys." *Pediatrics* 83, no. 1 (1989):7–17.

Kay, A., et al. "Hyposensitization for food-induced hyperkinetic syndrome." *Lancet* 341, no. 8837 (Jan 1993):114-115.

Latcham, F., et al. "A consistent pattern of minor immunodeficiency and subtle enteropathy in children with multiple food allergy." *Journal of Pediatrics* 143, no. 1 (Jul 2003):39–47.

Lucarelli, S., et al. "Food allergy and infantile autism." *Panminerva Medica* 37, no. 3 (Sep 1995):137–141.

Marshall, P. "Attention deficit disorder and allergy: A neurochemical model of the relation between the illnesses." *Psychological Bulletin* 106, no. 3 (Nov 1989):434–436.

McLoughlin, J.A. and M. Nall. "Teacher opinion of the role of food allergy on school behavior and achievement." *Annals of Allergy, Asthma and Immunology* 61 (1988):89–91.

Price, C., et al. "Associations of excessive irritability with common illnesses and food intolerance." *Paediatric and Perinatal Epidemiology* 4, no. 2 (Apr 1990):156–160.

Schaub, J. "Hyposensitization in children with food-induced hyperkinetic syndrome." *European Journal of Pediatrics* 151, no. 11 (Nov 1992):864–865.

Uhlig, T., et al. "Topographic mapping of brain electrical activity in children with food-induced attention deficit hyperkinetic disorder." *European Journal of Pediatrics* 156, no. 7 (Jul 1997):557–561.

Van, H., S. Jones, and M. Giacomantonio. "Food elimination based on IgG antibodies in irritable bowel syndrome: A randomized controlled trial." *Gut* 53, no. 10 (Oct 2004):1459–1464.

Step 8

Ashkenazi, A., S. Levin, and D. Krasilowsky. "Gluten and autism." *Lancet* 1, no. 8160 (Jan 19 1980):157.

Bowers, L. "An audit of referrals of children with autism spectrums disorder to the dietetic service." *Journal of Human Nutrition and Dietetics* 15, no. 2 (Apr 2002):141–144.

Christison, G. and K. Ivany. "Elimination diets in autism spectrum disorders: Any wheat amidst the chaff?" *Journal of Developmental and Behavioral Pediatrics* 27, no. 2 (Apr 2006):S162–171.

Cornish, E. "Gluten and casein free diets in autism: A study of the effects on food choice and nutrition." *Journal of Human Nutrition and Dietetics* 15, no. 4 (Aug 2002):261–269.

Dochniak, M. "Autism spectrum disorders—Exogenous protein insult." *Medical Hypotheses* 69, no. 3 (2007):545–549.

Elder, J., et al. "The gluten-free, casein-free diet in autism: Results of a preliminary double blind clinical trial." *Journal of Autism and Development Disorder* 36, no. 3 (Apr 2006):413–420.

George, V. and N. Wellman. "Meal time teams at work: Promoting nutrition goals in the individual education plan." *Journal of Nutrition Education* 33, no. 1 (Jan–Feb 2001):61–62.

Hadjivassiliou, M., et al. "Wheat protein can trigger severe headaches." *Neurology* 56 (2001):385–388.

Jyonouchi, H., et al. "Evaluation of an association between gastrointestinal symptoms and cytokine production against common dietary proteins in children with autism spectrum disorders." *Journal of Pediatrics* 146, no. 5 (May 2005):582–584.

————. "Dysregulated innate immune responses in young children with autism spectrum disorders: Their relationship to gastrointestinal symptoms and dietary intervention." *Neuropsychobiology* 51 (2005):77–85.

————. "Proinflammatory and regulatory cytokine production associated with innate and adaptive immune responses in children with autism spectrum disorders and developmental regression." *Journal of Neuroimmunology* 120 (2001):170–179.

Jyonouchi, H. "Innate immunity associated with inflammatory responses and cytokine production against common dietary proteins in patients with autism spectrum disorder." *Neuropsychobiology* 46, no. 2 (2002):76–84.

Kavale, K and S. Forness. "Hyperactivity and diet treatment: A meta-analysis of the Feingold hypothesis." *Journal of Learning Disabilities* 16, no. 6 (Jun–Jul 1983):324–330.

Knivsberg, A., et al. "A randomized, controlled study of dietary intervention in autistic syndromes." *Nutritional Neuroscience* 5, no. 4 (Sep 2002):251–261.

Knivsberg, A., K. Reichelt, and M. Nodland. "Reports on dietary intervention in autistic disorders." *Nutritional Neuroscience* 4, no. 1 (2001):25–37.

Lucarelli, S., et al. "Food allergy and infantile autism." *Panminerva Medica* 37, no. 3 (Sep 1995):137–141.

McCarthy, D. and M. Coleman. "Response of intestinal mucosa to gluten challenge in autistic subgroup." *Lancet* 2, no. 8148 (Oct 27 1979):877–878.

McCary, J. "Improving access to school-based nutrition services for children with special health care needs." *Journal of the American Dietetic Association* 106, no. 9 (Sep 2006):1333–1336.

Mercer, M. and M. Holder. "Food cravings, endogenous opioid peptides, and food intake: A review." *Appetite* 29, no. 3 (Dec 1997):325–352.

Milward, C., et al. "Gluten- and casein-free diets for autistic spectrum disorder." *Cochrane Database Systems Review* 2 (2004):CD003498.

Pavone, L., et al. "Autism and celiac disease: Failure to validate the hypothesis that a link might exist." *Biological Psychiatry* 42, no. 1 (Jul 1997):72–75.

Reichelt, K. and A. Knivsberg. "Can the pathophysiology of autism be explained by the nature of the discovered urine peptides?" *Nutritional Neuroscience* 6, no. 1 (Feb 2003):19–28.

Reichelt, K., et al. "Nature and consequences of hyperpeptiduria and bovine casomorphins found in autistic syndromes." *Developmental Brain Dysfunction* 7 (1994):71–85.

————. "Gluten, milk proteins and autism. Dietary intervention effects on behavior and peptide secretion." *Journal of Applied Nutrition* 42 (1990):1–11.

Rimland, B. "The Feingold diet: An assessment of the reviews by Mattes, by Kavale and Forness and others." *Journal of Learning Disabilities* 16, no. 6 (Jun–Jul 1983):331–333.

Shattock, P. and P. Whiteley. "Biochemical aspects in autism spectrum disorders: Updating the opioid-excess theory and presenting new opportunities for biomedical intervention." *Expert Opinions on Therapeutic Targets* 6, no. 2 (Apr 2002):175–183.

Shattock, P. and G. Lowdon. "Proteins, peptides and Autism Part 2: Implications for the education and care of people with autism." *Brain Dysfunction* 4 (1991):323–334.

Shattock, P., et al. "Role of neuropeptides in autism and their relationships with classical neurotransmitter." *Brain Dysfunction* 3 (1990):328.

Shaw W, et al. "Increased excretion of analogs of krebs cycle metabolites and arabinose in two brothers with autistic features." *Clinical Chemistry* 41 (1995):1094–1104.

Starobrat-Hermelin, B., et al. "The effects of magnesium physiological supplementation on hyperactivity in children with attention deficit hyperactivity disorder: Positive response to magnesium oral loading test." *Magnesium Research* 10, no. 2 (Jun 1997):149–156.

Vojdani, A., et al. "Antibodies to neuron-specific antigens in children with autism: Possible cross-reaction with encephalitogenic proteins from milk, Chlamydia pneumoniae, and streptococcus group A." *Journal of Neuroimmunology* 129 (2002):168–177.

Whiteley, P. "A gluten-free diet as an intervention for autism and associated spectrum disorders: Preliminary findings." *Autism* 3, no. 1 (1999):45–65.

Zhongjie, S., et al. "B-casomorphin induces Fos-like immunoreactivity in discrete brain regions relevant to schizophrenia and autism." *Autism* 3, no. 1 (1999):67–83.

———. "A peptide found in schizophrenia and autism causes behavioral changes in rats." *Autism* 3, no. 1 (1999):85–95.

Step 9

Bernstein, A. "Vitamin B$_6$ in clinical neurology." *Annals of the New York Academy of Science* 585 (1990):250–260.

Burd, L., et al. "A 15-year follow-up of a body with pyridoxine (vitamin B$_6$) dependent seizures with autism, breath holding, and severe mental retardation." *Journal of Child Neurology* 15, no. 11 (Nov 2000):763–765.

Findling R, et al. "High-dose pyridoxine and magnesium administration in children with autistic disorder: An absence of salutary effects in a double-blind, placebo-controlled study." *Journal of Autism and Developmental Disorders* 27, no. 4 (Aug 1997):467–478.

Food and Nutrition Board, Institute of Medicine, National Academies. Dietary Reference Intakes for Calcium, Phosphorous, Magnesium, Vitamin D, and Fluoride (1997).

———. Recommended Daily Allowance for Vitamin B$_6$. (2004).

Kleijnen, J. and P. Knipschild. "Niacin and vitamin B$_6$ in mental functioning: A review of controlled trials in humans." *Biological Psychiatry* 29, no. 9 (May 1991):931–941.

Kuriyama, S., et al. "Pyridoxine treatment in a subgroup of children with pervasive developmental disorders." *Developmental Medicine & Child Neurology* 44 (2002). 283–286.

Lelord, G., E. Callaway, and J. Muh. "Clinical and biological effects of high does of vitamin B$_6$ and magnesium on autistic children." *Acta Vitaminol Enzymol* 4, no. 1–2 (1982):27–44.

Lelord, G., et al. "Effects of pyridoxine and magnesium on autistic symptoms—initial observations." *Journal of Autism and Developmental Disorders* 11, no. 2 (Jun 1981):219–230.

Lerner v, et al. "Vitamin B_6 as add-on treatment in chronic schizophrenic and schizoaffective patients: A double-blind, placebo-controlled study." *Journal of Clinical Psychiatry* 63, no.1 (Jan 2002);54–58.

Martineau, J., et al. "Electrophysiological effects of fenfluramine or combined vitamin B_6 and magnesium on children with autistic behavior." *Developmental Medicine and Child Neurology* 31, no. 6 (Dec 1989):721–727.

———. "Brief report: An open middle-term study of combined vitamin B_6-magnesium in a subgroup of autistic children elected on their sensitivity to this treatment." *Journal of Autism and Developmental Disorders* 18, no. 3 (Sep 1988):435–447.

———. "Vitamin B6, magnesium, and combined B_6-Mg: Therapeutic effects in childhood autism." *Biological Psychiatry* 20, no. 5 (May 1985):467–478.

———. "Effects of vitamin B_6 on averaged evoked potentials in infantile autism." *Biological Psychiatry* 16, no.7 (Jul 1981):627–641.

Martineau, J., C. Barthelemy, and G. Lelord. "Long-term effects of combined vitamin B_6-magnesium administration in an autistic child." *Biological Psychiatry* 21, no. 5–6 (May 1986):511–518.

Menage, P., et al. "CD4+ CD45RA+ T lymphocyte deficiency in autistic children: Effect of a pyridoxine-magnesium treatment." *Brain Dysfunction* 5 (1992):326–333.

Mousain-Bosc, M., et al. "Improvement of neurobehavioral disorders in children supplemented with magnesium-vitamin B_6: Pervasive developmental disorder-autism." *Magnesium Research* 19, no. 1 (Mar 2006):53–62.

———. "Improvement of neurobehavioral disorders in children supplemented with magnesium-vitamin B_6: Attention deficit hyperactivity disorders." *Magnesium Research* 19, no. 1 (Mar 2006):46–52.

———. "Magnesium VitB_6 intake reduces central nervous system hyperexcitability in children." *Journal of the American College of Nutrition* 23, no. 5 (Oct 2004):545S–548S.

Nye, C. and A. Brice. "Combined vitamin B_6—magnesium treatment in autism spectrum disorder." *Cochrane Database System Review* 19, no. 4 (Oct 2005):CD003497.

———. "Combined vitamin B_6—magnesium treatment in autism spectrum disorder." *Cochrane Database System Review*, no. 4 (2002):CD003497.

Pfeiffer, S., et al. "Efficacy of vitamin B_6 and magnesium in the treatment of autism: A methodology review and summary of outcomes." *Journal of Autism and Developmental Disorders* 25, no. 5 (Oct 1995):481–493.

Rimland, B. "High dose vitamin B_6 and magnesium in treating autism: Response to study by Findling et al." *Journal of Autism and Developmental Disorders* 28, no. 6 (Dec 1998):581–582.

————. "Critique of "Efficacy of vitamin B$_6$ and magnesium in the treatment of autism." *Journal of Autism and Developmental Disorders* 28, no. 6 (Dec 1998):580–581.

————. "Controversies in the treatment of autistic children: Vitamin and drug therapy." *Journal of Child Neurology* 3 (1988):S68–72.

Rimland, B., E. Callaway, and P. Dreyfus. "The effects of high doses of vitamin B$_6$ on autistic children: A double-blind crossover study." *American Journal of Psychiatry* 135, no. 4 (Apr 1978):472–475.

Tolbert, L., et al. "Brief report. lack of response in an autistic population to a low dose clinical trial of pyridoxine plus magnesium." *Journal of Autism and Developmental Disorders* 23, no. 1 (Mar 1993):193–199.

Step 10

Adriani, W., et al. "Acetyl-L-carnitine reduces impulsive behavior in adolescent rats." *Psychopharmacology (Berl)* 176, no. 3–4 (Nov 2004):296–304.

Akhondzadeh, S., et al. "Zinc sulfate as an adjunct to methylphenidate for the treatment of attention deficit hyperactivity disorder in children: A double blind and randomized trial." *BMC Psychiatry* (Apr 8 2004):9.

Alberti, A., et al. "Sulphation deficit in 'low-functioning' autistic children: A pilot study." *Biological Psychiatry* 46 (1999):420–424.

Arnold, L. "Alternative treatments for adults with attention-deficit hyperactivity disorder (ADHD)." *Annals of the New York Academy of Science* 931 (Jun 2001):310–341.

Arnold, L., et al. "Serum zinc correlates with parent and teacher rated inattention in children with attention deficit/hyperactivity disorder." *Journal of Child Adolescent Psychopharmacology* 15, no. 4 (Aug 2005):628–636.

Ashwood, P., S. Wills, and J. Van de Water. "The immune response in autism: A new frontier for autism research." *Journal of Leukocyte Biology* 80, no. 1 (Jul 2006):1–15.

Bagchi, D., et al. "Protective effects of grape seed proanthocyanidins and selected antioxidants against TPA-induced hepatic and brain lipid peroxidation and DNA fragmentation, and peritoneal macrophage activation in mice." *General Pharmacology* 30 (1988):771–776.

Ballatoari, N., M. Lieberman, and W. Wang. "N-acetylcysteine as an antidote in methylmercury poisoning." *Environmental Health Perspectives* 106 (1998):267–271.

Bolman W. and J. Richmond. "A double-blind, placebo-controlled, crossover pilot trial of low dose dimethylglycine in patients with autistic disorder." *Journal of Autism and Developmental Disorders* 29, no. 3 (Jun 1999):191–194.

Chez, M., et al. "Double-blind, placebo-controlled study of L-carnosine supplementation in children with autistic spectrum disorders." *Journal of Child Neurology* 17, no. 11 (Nov 2002). 833–837.

Cohly, H. and A. Panja. "Immunological findings in autism." *International Review of Neurobiology* 71 (2005):317–341.

Dolske, M., et al. "A preliminary trial of ascorbic acid as supplemental therapy for autism." *Progress on Neuro-psychopharmacol and Biological Psychiatry* 17, no. 5 (Sep 1993):765–774.

Dosman, C., et al. "Children with autism: Effect of iron supplementation on sleep and ferritin." *Pediatric Neurology* 36, no. 3 (Mar 2007):152–158.

————. "Ferritin as an indicator of suspected iron deficiency in children with autism spectrum disorder: Prevalence of low serum ferritin concentration." *Developmental Medicine and Child Neurology* 48, no. 12 (Dec 2006):1008–1009.

Ellaway, C., et al. "Rett Syndrome: Randomized controlled trial of L-carnitine." *Journal of Child Neurology* 14 (1999):162–167.

Grimaldi, B. "The central role of magnesium deficiency in Tourette's syndrome: Causal relationships between magnesium deficiency, altered biochemical pathways and symptoms relating to Tourette's syndrome, and several reported comorbid conditions." *Medical Hypotheses* 58, no. 1 (Jan 2002):47–60.

Hallberg, L. "Search for nutritional confounding factors in the relationship between iron deficiency and brain function." *American Journal of Clinical Nutrition* 50 (1989):598–606.

James, S., P. Cutler, and S. Melnyks. "Metabolic biomarkers of increased oxidative stress and impaired methylation capacity in children with autism." *American Journal of Clinical Nutrition* 80 (2004):1611–1617.

Hendler, S. and D. Rorvik. *PDR for Nutritional Supplements* (1st ed). Thomson Healthcare, 2001.

Kern, J., et al. "Effectiveness of N, N-dimethylglycine in autism and pervasive development disorder." *Journal of Child Neurology* 16, no. 3 (Mar 2001):169–173.

Kidd, P. "Autism, an extreme challenge to integrative medicine, Part 2: medical management." *Alternative Medicine Review* 7, no. 6 (Dec 2002):472–499.

Konofal, E., et al. "Effectiveness of iron supplementation in a young child with attention-deficit/hyperactivity disorder." *Pediatrics* 116, no. 5 (Nov 2005):e732–734.

Konofal, E., et al. "Iron supplementation may help children with ADHD." *Archives of Pediatric and Adolescent Medicine* 158, no. 12 (Dec 2004):1113–1115.

Kozielec, T. and B. Starobrat-Hermelin. "Assessment of magnesium levels in children with attention deficit hyperactivity disorder (ADHD)." *Magnesium Research* 10, no. 2 (Jun 1997):143–148.

Lowe, T., et al. "Folic acid and B12 in autism and neuropsychiatric disturbances of childhood." *Journal of the American Academy of Child and Adolescent Psychiatry* 20, no. 1 (Winter 1981):104–111.

McGinnis, W. "Oxidative stress in autism." *Alternative Therapies in Health and Medicine* 10, no. 6 (Nov–Dec 2004):22–36; quiz 37, 92.

Megson, M. "Is autism a G-alpha protein defect reversible with natural vitamin A?" *Medical Hypotheses* 54, no. 6 (Jun 2000);979–983.

Nutrient Data Laboratory, United States Department of Agriculture. USDA National Nutrient Database for Standard Reference. Available at http://www.nal.usda.gov/fnic/food-comp.

Oudheusden, V. and H. Scholte. "Efficacy of carnitine in the treatment of children with attention-deficit hyperactivity disorder." *Prostaglandins, Leukotrienes and Essential Fatty Acids* 67, no. 1 (Jul 2002):33.

O'Reilly, B. and R. Waring. "Enzyme and sulphur oxidation deficiencies in autistic children with known food/chemical intolerance." *Journal of Orthomolecular Medicine* 8 (1993):198–200.

Pollitt, E., et al. "Iron deficiency and cognitive test performance in preschool children." *Nutrition and Behavior* 1 (1983):137–146.

Quinn, P., et al. "Carnosine: Its properties, functions, and potential therapeutic applications." *Molecular Aspects of Medicine* 13, no. 5 (1992):379–444.

Schneider, C., et al. "Oral human immunoglobulin for children with autism and gastrointestinal dysfunction: A prospective, open-label study." *Journal of Autism and Developmental Disorders* 36, no. 8 (Nov 2006):1053–1064.

Starobrat-Hermelin, B., et al. "The effects of magnesium physiological supplementation on hyperactivity in children with attention deficit hyperactivity disorder: Positive response to magnesium oral loading test." *Magnesium Research* 10, no. 2 (Jun 1997):149–156.

Stern, L., et al. "Immune function in autistic children." *Annals of Allergy, Asthma and Immunology* 95, no. 6 (Dec 2005):558–565.

Tarnha, M., et al. "Hydroxyl radical scavenging by carnosine and Cu(ii)-carnosine complexes." *International Journal of Radiation Biology* 75, no. 9 (1999):1177–1188.

Thomson Healthcare. *PDR for Herbal Medicines* (4th ed). Thomson Reuters, 2007.

Torrioli, M., et al. "Double-blind, placebo-controlled study of L-acetylcarnitine for the treatment of hyperactive behavior in fragile X syndrome." *American Journal of Medical Genetics* 87, no. 4 (Dec 1999):366–368.

Van Oudheusden, L. and H. Scholte. "Efficacy of carnitine in the treatment of children with attention-deficit hyperactivity disorder." *Prostaglandins, Leukotrienes and Essential Fatty Acids* 67, no.1 (Jul 2002):33–38.

Weber, W. and S. Newmark. "Complementary and alternative medical therapies for attention-deficit/hyperactivity disorder and autism." *Pediatric Clinics of North America* 54, no. 6 (Dec 2007):983–1006.

Yorbik, O., et al. "Potential effects of zinc on information processing in boys with attention deficit hyperactivity disorder." *Progress in Neuro-psychopharmacology and Biological Psychiatry* (Nov 17 2007). Epub ahead of print.

INDEX

Acetylcholine, 130, 241, 247

Acetylcholinesterase, 16, 241

Adequate Intake (AI), 34, 35, 37, 41, 55–56, 130, 222–224, 243

Adrenaline, 18, 241, 248

Aggression
    and data collection forms, 234, 235, 236
    and medication, 67
    and neurotoxins, 2, 139
    and omega-3 fatty acids, 52
    and serotonin, 120, 249
    and sugar, 18

AIDS, 119

Airborne allergies, 97–98, 101, 102

Allergens, 245
    airborne, 98
    and cross contamination, 242
    defined, 241
    and food allergies, 92, 94, 97, 98, 100, 111, 244, 245
    and supplements, 45, 46
    See also Food allergies

Alpha-linolenic acid (ALA), 23, 53, 55–56, 60, 243

Alpha-lipoic acid, 139, 140, 239, 240

Alpha-tocopherol, 138, 241

American Academy of Pediatrics (AAP), 130

American Dietetic Association (ADA), 213, 214, 215

Amino acids, ix, 140, 239
    and brain, 1, 13, 24, 26
    and carnitine, 129
    essential, 23, 25, 109, 129, 241, 242, 245, 248
    and GI health and disorders, 2, 86, 87
    and peptides, 104, 244

    and protein, 24, 25, 26, 86, 95, 109, 241, 242, 243, 245, 248
    purposes of, 24
    and supplements, 128, 141, 142
    and vitamins and minerals, 33
    See also particular amino acids

Anal fissures, 66, 241

Anaphylaxis, 92, 241

Antifungal Diet, 3, 103, 114–115

Antifungals, 84, 85, 100, 114, 133, 241

Antioxidants, ix, 46, 128, 129, 131, 136, 137, 138, 140, 141, 142, 242, 247, 250

Applesauce muffins, 158

Applied Behavior Analysis (ABA), 47

Arachidonic acid (ARA), 15, 59

Arsenic, 1, 139, 238

Art therapy, x, xi

Artificial additives, 1, 9–14, 147
    colors, 10–11, 13, 20, 45, 46, 95, 115, 116, 238, 242
    flavors, 10, 11–12, 13, 20, 21, 45, 46, 95, 115, 116, 238
    and food sensitivities, 94–95, 115
    and gluten, casein, and soy, 106, 109, 110, 111
    preservatives, 10, 12–13, 20, 21, 95, 115, 238
    sweeteners, 10, 13–14, 20, 21, 95, 241

Aspartame, 13, 14, 21, 94, 115, 241

Aspartic acid, 13, 241

Asperger's Syndrome, ix
    and dietitians, 215
    and food allergies, 91
    and nutrition, x, 2
    and supplements, 48

Aspiration, 64, 68, 241

Aspirin, 115

Food Chaining, 73–74

Food Chaining: The Proven 6-Step Plan to Stop Picky Eating, Solve Feeding Problems, and Expand Your Child's Diet (Fraker, Walbert, Cox, and Fishbein), 74

Food intolerance, 2, 66, 87, 92, 93, 95, 96, 232

Food protein–induced enterocolitis, 93, 244

Food sensitivity, 26, 66, 80, 87, 92, 93, 94–95, 96, 115, 232

Fraker, Cheri, 73, 74

French toast, 162

Fructose, 18, 21, 27, 86, 88, 95, 113, 245, 249

Fruit gelatin, 180

Gastric-emptying study, 66, 88, 244

Gastritis, 79, 244

Gastroenteritis, 93, 244

Gastroesophageal Reflux Disease (GERD), 64, 65, 82, 88, 89

Gastrointestinal (GI) disorders, ix, 44

   and autism, 2, 29, 42, 64–66, 79–90, 95–96, 99, 100, 104–105, 113, 241

   and behavior, 81–82

   and dietary treatment, 83–88, 103, 104, 105, 113–114, 114–115, 116

   and elimination problems, 80–81

   factors in, 82–83

   and feeding problems, 64–66, 80, 82

   and fiber, 29, 100

   and food allergies, 65, 66, 87–88, 93, 99, 100, 104

   and medical treatment, 88–89

   and nutrition therapy, 3, 99, 100

   symptoms, 79, 86, 87, 89–90

   and vitamin B_{12}, 143

Gastrointestinal (GI) system, x, 2, 22, 32, 37

Generally recognized as safe (GRAS), 9, 11, 14, 244

Gingerbread men, 177

Gliadomorphine, 104, 105, 244

Glossitis, 143, 244

Glucose, 245, 247

   and carbohydrates, 27–28, 29, 30, 245, 248

   and digestive enzymes, 86

   and magnesium, 120

   oxidation, 1, 244

   and protein, 24, 26

   and sugar, 18, 19, 113, 249

   and vitamin B_6, 121

   and vitamin D, 138

Glutamate, 11, 87, 141, 244, 247

Glutamic acid, 11, 244

Glutamine, 86, 87, 100, 241

Glutathione, 139, 140, 141, 239, 244, 248

Gluten, 45, 93, 103, 104, 105, 106–108, 110–112, 147

   See also Gluten Free Casein Free (GFCF) Diet

Gluten Free Casein Free (GFCF) Diet, 3, 4, 44, 46, 88, 103–113, 116–118, 134, 147–210, 228, 232

Glycemic index, 27–28, 245

Graham cracker–style cookies, 189

Granola, 163

Haas, Dr. Sydney, 113

Hamburger buns, 155

HDL, 15, 31

Herbicides, 139

Herbs, ix, 45

   and antifungals, 85

   and autism, x, 4, 128

   and detoxification, 238, 240

   and dietitians, 215

High-fructose corn syrup (HFCS), 18, 21, 27, 245

Hippotherapy, x, xi, 245

Histamine, 92, 96, 245, 247

Homocysteine, 245

Hot chocolate, 148

Hotdog rolls, 155

Hydrogen breath test, 245

Hydrogenation, 14, 245, 247

Hyperactivity, 124

   and artificial food additives, 10, 115

   and carnosine, 142

   and data collection forms, 234, 235, 236

   and diets, 105

   and food allergies, 96, 99, 101

   and medication, 67

   and neurotoxins, 2, 139

   and nutrition, 2